BEAUTY REWIND

BOOKS BY TAYLOR CHANG-BABAIAN

Asian Faces

Style Eyes

Beauty Rewind

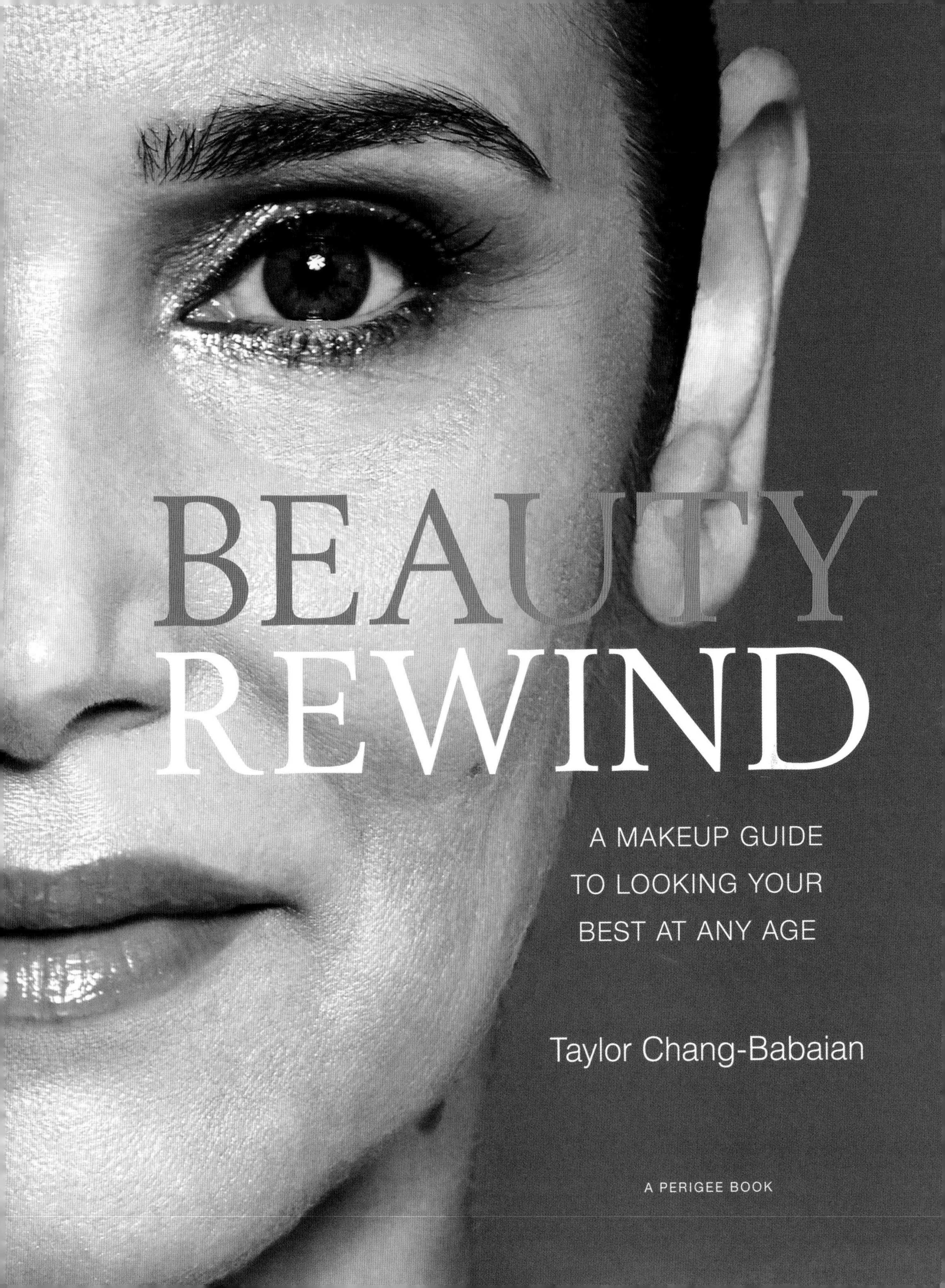

BEAUTY REWIND

A MAKEUP GUIDE
TO LOOKING YOUR
BEST AT ANY AGE

Taylor Chang-Babaian

A PERIGEE BOOK

A PERIGEE BOOK
Published by the Penguin Group
Penguin Group (USA) LLC
375 Hudson Street, New York, New York 10014

USA · Canada · UK · Ireland · Australia · New Zealand · India · South Africa · China

penguin.com

A Penguin Random House Company

BEAUTY REWIND

ISBN: 978-0-399-16305-0

First edition: October 2014

PRINTED IN THE UNITED STATES OF AMERICA

10   9   8   7   6   5   4   3   2   1

Text design by Pauline Neuwirth

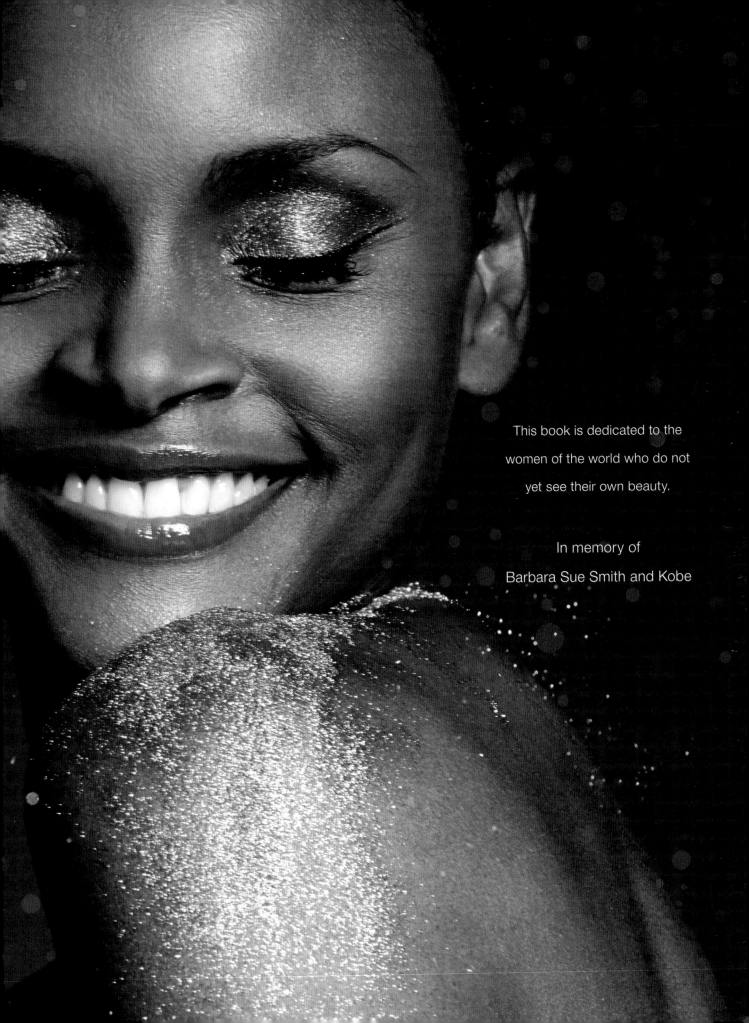

This book is dedicated to the women of the world who do not yet see their own beauty.

In memory of
Barbara Sue Smith and Kobe

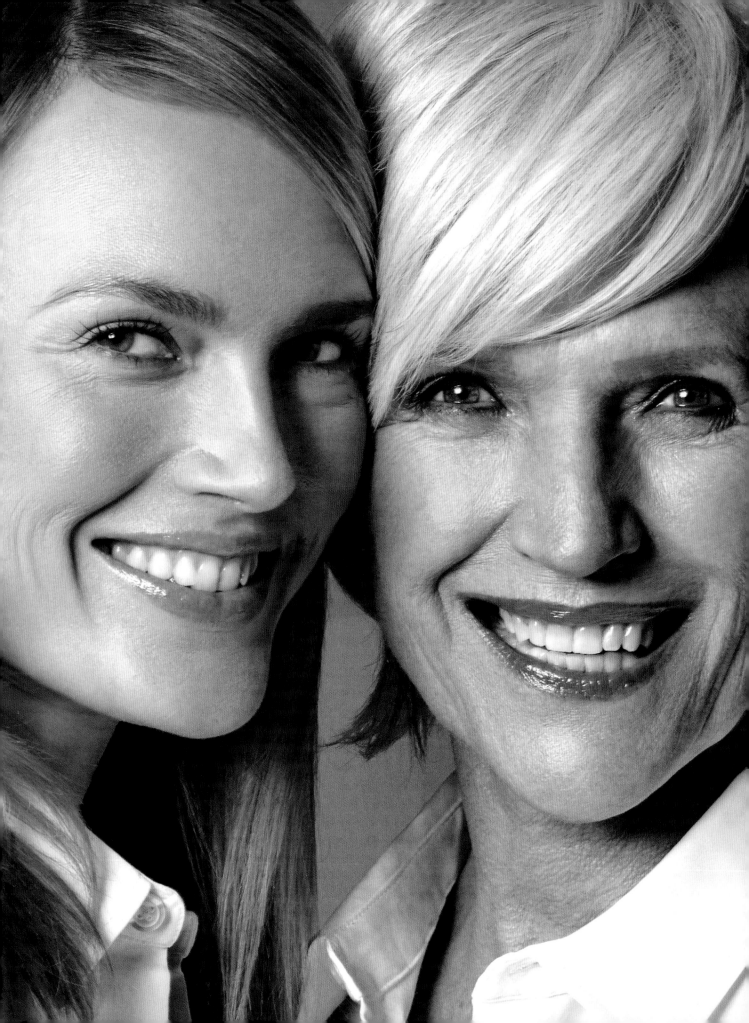

CONTENTS

They say that age is all in your mind. The trick is keeping it from creeping down into your body.

—Anonymous

INTRODUCTION

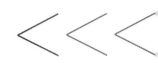

t's time that we change our attitudes about aging. It's going to happen to us, whether we complain about it or decide to live our best, most beautiful life. Getting older is a gift; not everyone gets to do it. Personally, I wouldn't trade my life today to be in my twenties again for anything. Besides, in our current beauty world, you have choices. You can slow down the appearance of aging by simply changing some daily habits, and look younger by adding a little color to your makeup routine.

Beauty Rewind is a detailed guide to addressing your concerns about aging: what causes it, how to prevent it from happening prematurely, how to correct or camouflage it naturally or aggressively, the best products to enhance your skin, the makeup looks that age you, and how to use makeup and current antiaging technology to look as young as you feel. Whether you're in your late twenties or eighties, I will give you the knowledge to help you look your best at any age.

This book is packed with advice I've collected in my twenty-plus years in the beauty industry. So whether you want to recapture your image from ten years ago (before your eyelids started drooping), emphasize your best features now, or just learn how to get rid of the sleep creases on your face before you get to work, then read ahead. And yes, in true Taylor fashion, you'll learn how to apply a smokey eye that even the young girls will envy.

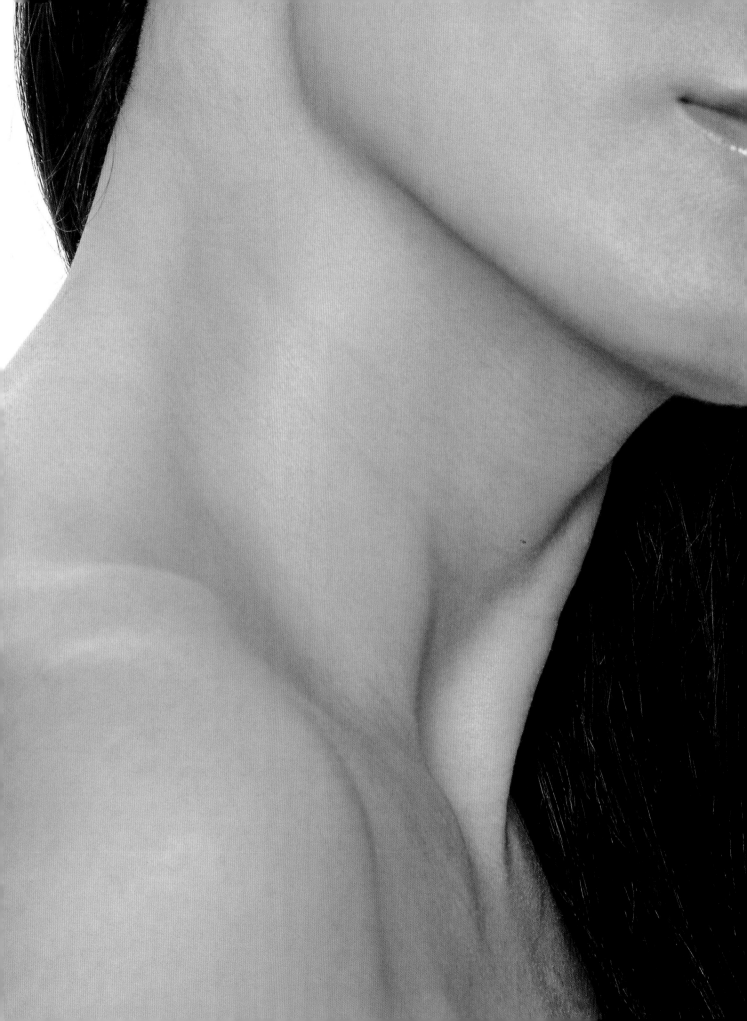

BEAUTY SCHOOL

From Skin-Care Basics to the Latest in Antiaging Technology

Aging happens to us all. But have you noticed some women seem to age better than others? I've seen some fortysomethings look like they're in their late twenties, while others look like they're in their fifties. We all age at various rates; the trick is to slow that rate down as much as possible and enhance the features we love. Sometimes aging well is genetic, but even good genes will only take you so far. As a makeup artist, I feel truly blessed to have met and worked with thousands of women—real women who don't have on-call dermatologists and celebrity makeup artists, or referrals to the next big plastic surgeon. As they get older, many women who have never worn makeup all of a sudden feel like they need a little help.

GENETICS AND SKIN

They say you can always tell what a woman will look like as she ages if you look at her mother. That's only partly true. Genes do play a role in how we age. They determine how you make proteins and collagen, which gives skin its strength, and they're also why some women age faster than others. Genetics also play a role in whether your skin will tend to freckle, wrinkle, or sag first when aging. Thankfully, however, your daily habits—how you take care of your body and skin—will be the most important factor in how you age.

PREMATURE AGING

Genes also determine skin color, which is a huge factor in how you are affected by elements in the environment, such as sunlight. While there are several contributors

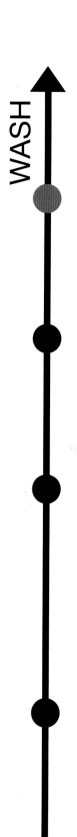

WASH

to premature aging, stress, environmental factors, smoking, and the sun are the biggest. The number one cause of premature aging is the sun's UVA and UVB rays, which break down our skin. As we age, several things happen to our skin that can make us look older. Our skin gets thinner as it loses fatty tissue. The collagen breaks down, causing our face to sag. We produce less oil in our glands, which causes skin to become drier. We produce less melanin, which causes our skin color to become sallow and lose definition, as well as reduces our natural protection from environmental skin damage. Skin pigmentation or melanin acts as a natural sunscreen. The lighter your skin, the more sensitive you are to sun damage. This does not mean that those with darker skin should not protect themselves. While the higher melanin content of darker skin gives some protection from the sun and protects the epidermis (the top layer), the underlying part of the dermis (inside layers) is still open to damage like lighter skin. The result is the breakdown of collagen, which causes skin to sag. This is why lighter skin tends to wrinkle earlier in the aging process, while darker skin tends to sag. Aging can happen at a rapid pace if you sit back and let it happen—or you can slow down the process by doing something about it.

Our lives are busier than ever, but taking care of your skin doesn't have to be difficult or complicated. A few minutes and four simple steps: washing, exfoliating, moisturizing, and protecting, will make a world of difference in how your skin ages.

THE DAILY FOUR

1. WASH

I know the last thing you want to do after a hard day is wash your face, but a clean face ensures you don't feed the bacteria on your skin. Dirty skin creates clogged pores and excess dead skin cells, which ultimately lead to aging skin. The key is to remove all difficult makeup prior to washing your face. This includes dark-colored lipsticks or glosses, as well as smudge-proof eye makeup such as eyeliners and mascaras. Doing this prior to washing will ensure a complete cleanse.

When using a foaming or gel cleanser, gently splash warm water on your face several times to loosen dirt and makeup. Use your fingers to rub in cleanser in a circular, upward motion; don't forget your jawline and harder-to-reach areas such as the sides of your nose. Avoid washing your face in an up-and-down vertical motion, which can pull on skin. Use warm water to rinse skin and repeat if necessary. In the morning, rinse skin with cool water (not cold water, as this could pop capillaries). Rinsing with cool water reduces swelling that can occur during sleep and wakes up the senses.

A favorite of women in the East and rapidly gaining popularity in the West, cleansing oils can be a great solution for sensitive as well as dry skin. Apply a pump of cleansing oil to your fingers and massage it into your face and neck in circular motions for a minimum of one minute, and rinse clean.

2. EXFOLIATE

We produce new skin about every twenty-eight days when we are young. As we age, that rate drastically reduces. We need to exfoliate, sloughing off old skin cells, to increase the rate at which new skin is produced. Exfoliating also removes excess dirt and oil, which your cleanser may not have picked up; this gives skin a fresher look, and also helps to shrink pores.

Exfoliate daily in the morning and evening, prior to moisturizing. Most exfoliants can be applied with a cotton pad; however, be certain to avoid the eye area. When using aggressive exfoliants like glycolic acid or Retin-A, use only during evening regimens, as sun exposure to fresh skin can accelerate skin damage. With all exfoliants, it is essential to wear a sunscreen with SPF 30-plus to protect the skin from harmful rays, which can be even more damaging to the newer skin.

FRUIT ENZYME: Derived from fruits such as papaya and pineapple, fruit enzyme exfoliants gently loosen the bonds that hold dead skin cells onto the surface. Great for exfoliating delicate, sensitive skin.

SALICYLIC ACID: A plant-based acid, which helps skin cell turnover. Works best for oily and acne-prone skin.

GLYCOLIC ACID: A sugar-based acid that's great for unclogging pores and removing dead cells that create dull-looking skin. Start with products containing 5 percent glycolic acid and increase to only those with a content of 10 percent if necessary. Chemical peels contain 20 percent to 70 percent glycolic acid, and should never be done at home.

RETINOL: Nonprescription-strength vitamin A derived from animals.

RETIN-A: A prescription-strength acid derivative of vitamin A. Also known as tretinoin, it is an aggressive exfoliant that can be used daily at home with the supervision of your doctor. Retin-A can cause peeling of the skin, which can make applying foundation difficult. Try cutting down usage to every other day should this occur and tap on foundation to prevent dead skin from rolling off, a sign that you may be applying too often.

EXFOLIATE

3. MOISTURIZE

Help keep skin moist by applying moisturizing products immediately after toweling off and exfoliating to provide the greatest absorption. Areas that don't have oil glands, such as the lips, or have minimal oil glands, such as the eye area, need special attention and require moisturizers made specifically for these areas.

Use a moisturizer with SPF in the morning and a treatment one in the evening. This can be a light one for normal to combination skin or a thicker version for dry or mature skin. Apply to the skin in circular motions, taking your time to massage it in. Don't forget to apply to the neck and chest, too. Look for moisturizers that contain antioxidants (such as vitamins C and E) to protect from free radicals (airborne agents that cause cellular damage).

HYDRATING TONER: While an exfoliant is also called a toner, the use of a hydrating toner is different, and should become part of your normal routine. Hydrating toner is a watery substance that you gently tap onto the face or apply with a cotton pad. It usually contains ingredients such as hyaluronic acid (binds water to cells), and creates a deep glow to the skin from within.

EYE CREAM: The skin around the eyes is incredibly thin—a fraction of the thickness of the rest of your skin. This is why signs of aging show first around the eyes as fine lines or crow's-feet. It's essential to treat the area from the brow to the cheekbone delicately. Apply eye cream before makeup, to ensure a smooth application, and again during your evening regimen before sleep, when skin renews itself (something to think about the next time you rub your eyes or decide to skip the eye cream).

SERUMS: Contain concentrated products (usually peptides and antioxidants) that help prevent future aging as well as correct skin damage.

PEPTIDES: Peptides are a chain of amino acids that act as messengers to cells, and tell the skin what to do. Peptides can tell cells to produce more collagen. Look for serums or moisturizers that contain peptides.

ANTIOXIDANTS: Antioxidants like vitamins A, C, and E are essential in destroying free radicals, which can damage skin.

Drink plenty of water to keep the skin's elasticity at its best.

MOISTURIZE

4. PROTECT

Sunscreen

It continues to amaze me that so many women today are willing to undergo drastic surgery for wrinkles but don't wear sunscreen. The sun is a major cause of wrinkles, dryness, and hyperpigmentation, the leading cause of premature aging. To protect the skin from its damaging rays, choose sunscreens with *broad-spectrum* protection (protects skin from both UVA and UVB rays) that have an SPF of at least 30. While UVB rays cause burning on the outer surface of our skin, UVA rays, whose damage you cannot see until it's too late, attack under the surface and break down collagen, which can cause the most amount of aging. Wear sunscreen year-round. You may not be exposed to UVB rays during the winter, but you can still be susceptible to a significant amount of damage from UVA rays.

I've heard women make the excuse that sunscreens are too heavy for their skin, or that they have no time to apply additional products. While sunscreens can also be found in foundations, you'll do yourself a favor by doubling up with a broad-spectrum sunscreen in addition to a foundation that contains SPF, which can be used as an additional physical sunblock as well. The earlier in life you start applying sunscreen, the more protection you'll get against premature aging.

Note: Sunscreens can contain agents that adhere better to the skin so you don't sweat them off. These sunscreens are often waterproof and can require additional effort to remove (yes, it's worth it). Use an exfoliating brush or repeat cleansing with your cleanser until all residue is off. Exfoliants are also a great way of removing any leftover excess sunscreen on the skin, but should not be used in lieu of a thorough washing.

Physical versus Chemical Sunblock

Sunscreens help protect our skin in different ways by either reflecting or absorbing the sun's rays before they can damage the skin. Physical sunscreens such as titanium dioxide or zinc oxide reflect and scatter rays away from the skin. They also cover the entire spectrum of the sun's rays but can often feel thick or have a pasty, white consistency. Chemical sunblocks absorb the rays, which is why you have to apply them fifteen minutes prior to sun exposure. Chemical sunscreens are usually less dense in texture and contain a variety of chemicals for the different rays. Sunscreens that contain both chemical and physical sunscreens are most popular because they offer consistency and protection.

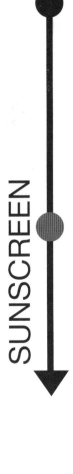

SUNSCREEN

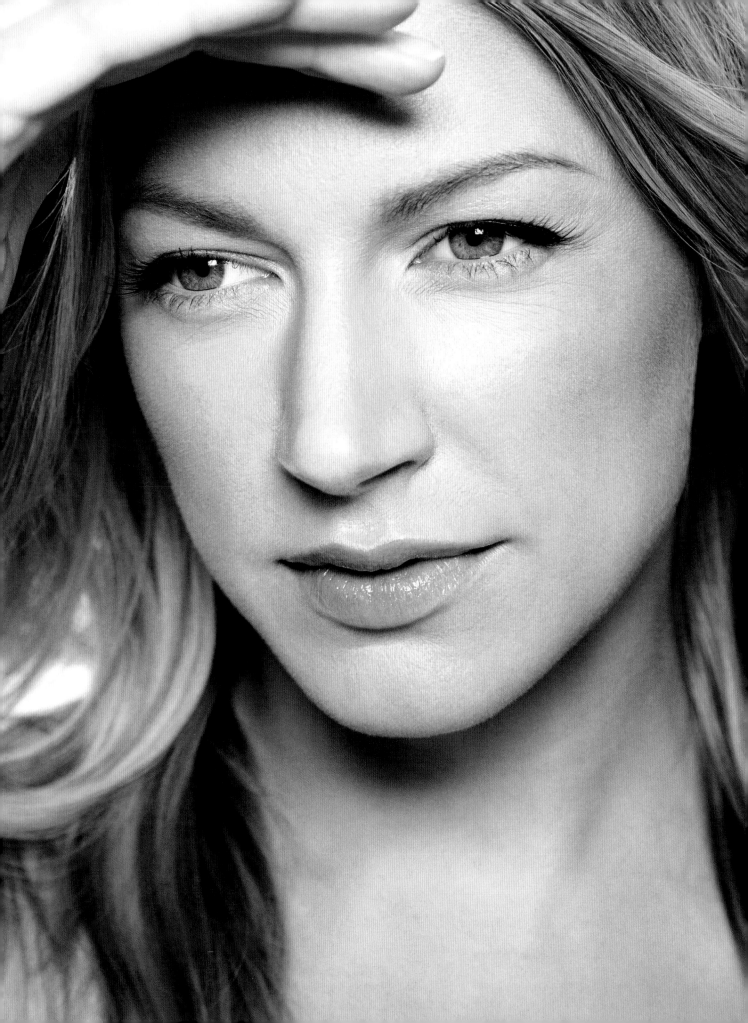

Quick Tips to Stay Safe in the Sun

- *Always wear sunscreen with a minimum SPF of 30-plus.*

- *Avoid being out in the sun from 10 a.m. to 3 p.m., especially during the summer.*

- *Cover skin with foundation to layer extra protection.*

- *Wear clothing and hats for additional protection.*

- *Wear sunglasses that protect the delicate eye area.*

- *Wear sunscreen even on overcast days, while driving, and while working indoors. Although you may not get burning rays, you can be exposed to aging rays from indoor lighting as well like fluorescents.*

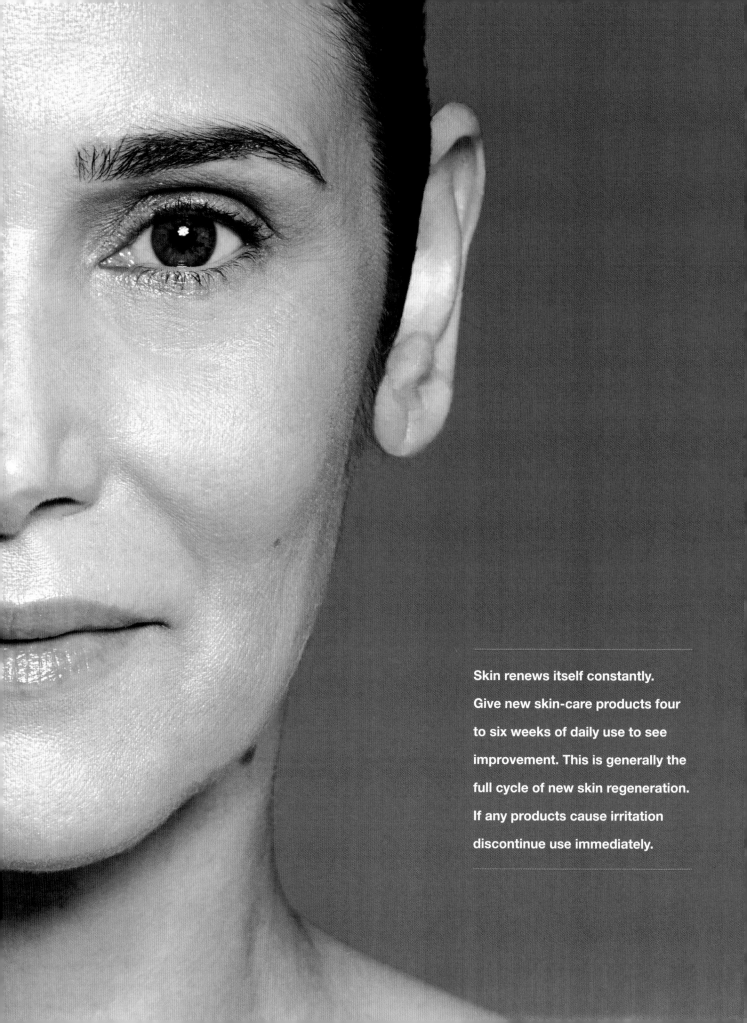

Skin renews itself constantly.
Give new skin-care products four
to six weeks of daily use to see
improvement. This is generally the
full cycle of new skin regeneration.
If any products cause irritation
discontinue use immediately.

GET NAKED

Removing all makeup, dirt, and environmental residue before bed is essential for the health and vitality of your skin as well as keeping skin appearing its most youthful. Leaving makeup on blocks pores, which can make them appear larger. By not removing makeup, dead cells and dirt accumulate, which can leave skin looking dull, a definite sign of aging skin. Not to mention skin renews itself when you're sleeping, which makes your evening skin-care regimen that much more important. Look for removers that are gentle, in order to protect delicate areas and prevent infections, which can be caused when dirt is left on the skin, allowing bacteria to multiply. Water is the most powerful cleansing agent. Combined with the right cleansing properties, it's your best way to clean your face. While makeup wipes are great temporary fixes and sometimes the only solution (that is, refreshing your makeup foundation before a night out), a good cleanser and warm water will give you the optimum result.

Put products, excluding cleansers, by the side of your bed to ensure that you do your routine at night. After an exhausting day it is more likely that you'll perform every step of your nighttime regimen if you are sitting in your bed rather than standing on your feet.

EYES

Washing the eye area ensures removal of any excess dirt, debris, and oil, allowing your eye creams to work properly and helps eyes stay healthy. When you don't remove your eye makeup thoroughly before bed, the body protects itself by flushing out excess debris and leaving discharge. This can be a sign that you're not cleansing the delicate eye area well enough, and can lead to possible infection. Between layers of concealer, eye shadow, eyeliner, and mascara, it's important to take all products off carefully to care for the health of your eyes. Look for oil-free, generally silicone-based removers that are meant specifically for the eye area. If you are using waterproof eye makeup (highly recommended for women going through menopause or just busy, active women as they don't smudge in the middle of the day and rarely need touching up), choose removers that are made specifically to remove waterproof cosmetics. Apply remover to a cotton pad, allow it to sit on the eyelids for a few seconds, and wipe away all eye makeup using a gentle touch. This should be quick and simple. The solution should not sting, and even with smokey eyes, all makeup should come off relatively easily. You can use a cotton swab to remove any excess in the hard-to-reach areas. Then continue with your regimen, washing your eye area and face with a gentle cleanser. If you are using a cleanser that contains any exfoliating properties such as salicylic acid, avoid the eye area and use a separate cleanser.

LIPS

To remove lipstick and lip gloss, use a clean tissue to wipe off as much product as possible first. If there is still any leftover stain, apply petroleum-based lip balm and let it sit for a few moments and then wipe off. While there are specific lipstick removers, eye makeup remover is a great alternative. This is essential to make sure there is no buildup around the lip line, which can cause irritations and blackheads. Use exfoliating scrubs such as sugar or a washcloth to gently exfoliate the skin and moisturize lips just as you would your skin, to help minimize shrinking.

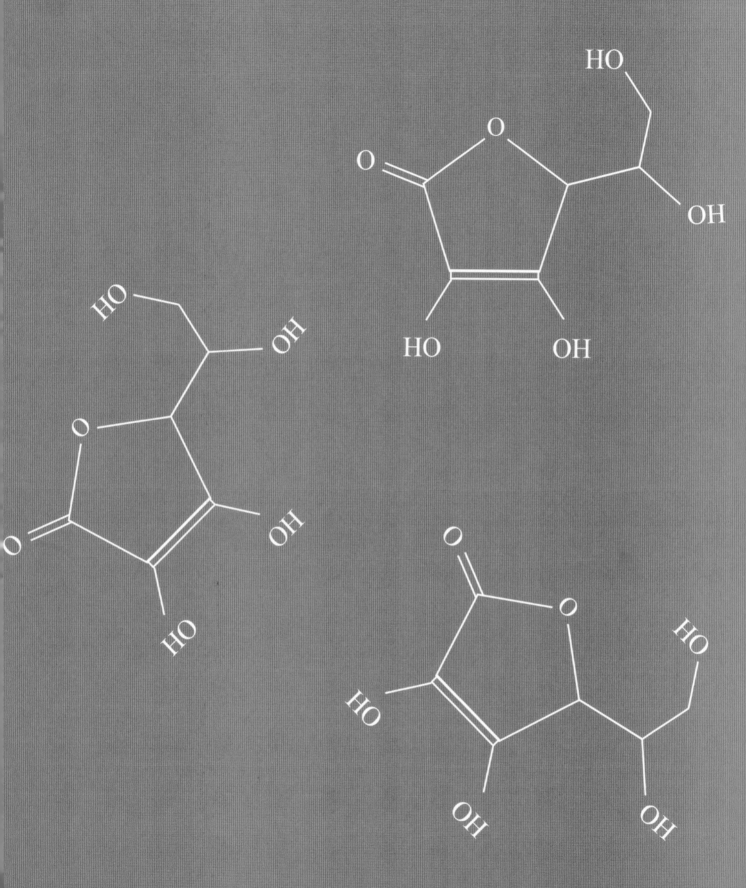

NEXT-LEVEL SKIN

At-Home and In-Office Care

It's important that before you partake in any aggressive skin-care solution, you first begin with a regimen of the *daily four* if you are not already doing so. Daily skin care can help minimize the appearance of aging skin and give you a better understanding of what aggressive procedure, if any, you really need. I have met far too many women who opted for Botox and Restylane, but, because they had no idea of basic skin care, were surprised six months later—after everything from the procedure had worn off—to find that their skin looked worse than before. Depending on the procedure, patients who rely only on treatments for skin upkeep in lieu of daily skin-care routines will discover that they need to incorporate a daily skin-care routine for the best results. Advanced chemical or technological procedures should continue where the daily regimen stops, not be a replacement. Maintain a daily skin-care regimen for at least sixty days to see optimal results.

Note: Before any in-office procedure make sure to notify your dermatologist about the products you are using at home.

AT HOME: OVER-THE-COUNTER SKIN TREATMENTS

MANUAL EXFOLIANTS

A handheld exfoliating device uses sonic technology to exfoliate the skin gently, and can be used in conjunction with your skin cleanser. The sonic frequency's rapid motion moves the brush gently back and forth up to three hundred times per second! These devices can be used daily or a few times a week to remove dead skin. They are perfect for removing excess makeup, dirt, oil, and sunscreen, and are reportedly six times more effective than cleanser alone. Exfoliating devices allow skin-care products to work more effectively because they leave the skin thoroughly clean, allowing products to better penetrate the skin. Avoid using in sensitive areas such as around the eyes and on open blemishes or cold sores.

KOJIC ACID

Made from a derivative of mushrooms, kojic acid inhibits the production of excess melanin in the skin. Often combined with hydroquinone and glycolic acid in products to fade hyperpigmentation.

HYDROQUINONE

Hydroquinone is a topical agent often found in low doses of around 2 percent in over-the-counter products used to prevent the overproduction of melanin. Though products with higher percentages of hydroquinone are available, they are not recommended because they can cause severe side effects like blotchy skin discoloration and irritation.

TRETINOIN/RETIN-A

One of the strongest topical exfoliants available with a dermatologist's prescription, tretinoin/Retin-A is excellent at rapid exfoliation of the skin to increase the rate of new skin growth and helps to rebuild collagen and reduce fine lines and hyperpigmentation. Apply only in the evenings, and use sunscreen generously in the mornings. During days of the year when UV rays can be high, like in summer, consider wearing extra protection or minimizing daily use of Retin-A as skin can thin and be more susceptible to damage, which will reverse any benefits.

SWEAT

Sweating is a great way to cleanse pores. Whether it's hitting the gym or the sauna, detoxify your pores often to keep them clean. It's best if you keep your pores clean of makeup when you sweat. If you prefer to wear cosmetics in the gym or out in the sun while working out, make sure the makeup is non-comedogenic and oil-free. After workouts, cleanse the skin properly to avoid clogging pores.

ANTIOXIDANTS

Antioxidants, including vitamin C, vitamin E, beta-carotene and vitamin A, help to minimize the aging process by reducing the effects of free radicals, which attach to healthy cells and cause cellular damage. Choose moisturizers containing antioxidants and eat antioxidant-rich foods such as berries, dark leafy green vegetables, and sweet potatoes. Vitamin C, in particular, is necessary to build collagen and help skin repair itself. Look for stable vitamin C serums to use prior to moisturizer and eat vitamin C–rich foods like sweet peppers, broccoli, and citrus fruits to maintain healthy skin. Skin-care products will include ingredients on the box or labels, though these may be listed by their chemical names—L-ascorbic acid (vitamin C), tocopheryl acetate (vitamin E), and retinyl palminate (vitamin A).

HYALURONIC ACID

A molecule made up of simple sugars, the body naturally produces hyaluronic acid to bind water to the skin and has the ability to hold up to one thousand times its weight in water. The body produces more hyaluronic acid, which gives skin its moisture, in younger years. Lucky for your aging skin, you can find hyaluronic acid as an ingredient in many moisturizers, serums, and hydrating toners. After application, hyaluronic acid gives the illusion of dewy, glowing skin.

SERUMS

Serums are products with a high concentration of various ingredients that penetrate deeper into the skin's surface, and should be an essential part of your skin-care routine as skin starts to age. Different serums are created for specific skin-care needs. You can find dark spot correctors and collagen builders as well as pore-refining blends. Seal in with moisturizer.

TREATMENT MASKS

Choose treatments depending on the needs of your skin, and use once or twice a week; this includes hydrating masks, which help plump dehydrated skin; clay masks to remove impurities or unclog pores; and retinol masks for fine lines and hyperpigmentation.

IN-OFFICE: DERMATOLOGIST TREATMENTS

Dermatologist-administered skin treatments can be an added weapon to combat aging skin. They can give you significantly faster results than over-the-counter treatments alone—at a price, of course. These treatments should only be in addition to proper skin care, however, not instead of. I've met numerous women who've had injections and aggressive medical procedures but who don't take care of their skin

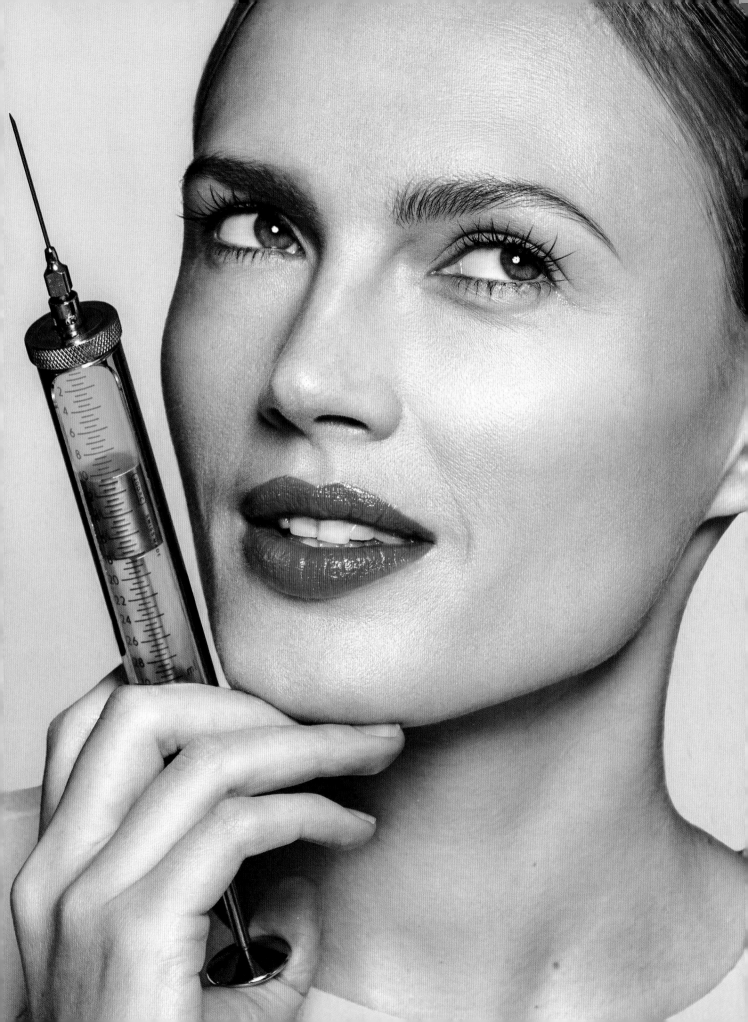

at home. These treatments correct the problems temporarily but once the injections wear off, the skin often looks worse than before. Making the decision of how extreme to take your skin-treatment regimen is a personal one. Whether you're looking for a more natural alternative or ready to take the dive into the peels or injections of extreme makeovers, it's important to research your options and your doctors, and really search your soul to find out what your true desires are.

COMMON ISSUES

Hyperpigmentation

Hyperpigmentation, an increase in melanin or dark patches on the skin, often occurs due to sun damage or a change in hormones, which can be caused by a number of factors such as aging, stress, medication, or pregnancy. You can prevent many instances of hyperpigmentation by using sunscreen. If you've experienced hyperpigmentation and already tried over-the-counter products, Retin-A or acid peels may be a good choice for you. Be sure to talk to your dermatologist to find out which treatment would work best for your skin.

Skin Tags

A skin tag is excess skin or tissue that hangs on the skin. These can usually be found near folds of skin and often occur when a person has excessive weight gain. Your dermatologist can perform a simple removal by cutting, freezing, or burning the tag off.

SURFACE RENEWAL

Microdermabrasion

This method uses very fine, rough grains to resurface the outer layer of the skin. Microdermabrasion causes the body to believe it is damaged and, thus, creates new skin. The finished product is a fresher-looking and better-feeling skin surface. This minimizes the appearance of fine lines and scarring, and allows skin-care products to better penetrate into the lower layers of the skin. Microdermabrasion only affects the epidermis of the skin and is good for ridding the outermost superficial skin of excess dead cells, which may otherwise be slow to come off. The procedure is also great for adding radiance to dull skin.

Chemical Peels

A stronger, more aggressive (but still noninvasive) treatment than microdermabrasion, chemical peels use acids (or a combination of various acids, depending on skin needs) to resurface the top layer of the skin. Chemical peels rejuvenate the surface of the skin by forcing cell renewal and rebuilding collagen and elasticity. They can be used to improve scarring, fine lines, and hyperpigmentation. Recovery time can take up to a few weeks, depending on the peel. Avoid sun exposure for at least a week prior to the peel and afterward.

After any skin procedure, always remember to wear sunscreen, avoid sun exposure, and cover up as much as possible with loose clothing.

Go Deeper

There are two types of fractional laser choices: ablative and non-ablative. The non-ablative, fractional laser therapy is a lower-intensity treatment that requires less down-time—usually one day—and can leave skin looking slightly sunburned and puffy. Non-ablative laser therapy generally requires three to four treatments to see the best results. A laser light that looks like several dots in a square format skips the epidermis and goes to the dermis, creating controlled damage. As the treated area heals, stronger, more youthful skin is created. In the past, laser resurfacing was often unsightly—patients looked like they were recovering from severe sunburn—and required as much as two to three weeks' recovery time. Advancements in technology have made the recovery much less unsightly. Fractional laser therapy can be a preemptive strike against needing a face-lift in in your sixties and is great for lines, firmness, spots, and dark skin. I recommend for those in their late thirties and beyond.

Fractional CO_2 laser is the ablative choice. It is a much more intensive treatment than fractional resurfacing. It is not for darker skin, as the treatment can cause discolored pigmentation. The required downtime is much longer due to the intensity of the treatment. Your skin can be unsightly for several days (similar to a burn) but you should be able to get back to work in a few weeks. Avoid the sun prior to the procedure and for about a month afterward as the fresh, new skin can be easily damaged.

Numbing cream is applied and left on to penetrate deeper into the layers of skin for up to an hour prior to the procedure. Protective eyewear is essential to protect corneas from lasers. CO_2 lasers go deep into skin, creating more aggressive controlled damage, which results in new collagen formations and more youthful skin.

Side effects may include pain, swelling, severe redness for several days, scabbing, hyperpigmentation, and scarring.

Anytime you are participating in aggressive treatments and you are taking any medications that can affect the outcome, it's important to stop prior to and between treatments. Avoid sun exposure before and after treatment, as the sun can harm new skin or make skin more sensitive to procedures. Darker skin with higher melanin content can grow back unevenly. Postpone treatment if you have any open sores, including acne and cold sores. Note that treatments can be painful and there is always a slight risk of infection, especially with ablative treatments. Talk to your dermatologist if you are more sensitive to pain or are taking any medications including over-the-counter ones. Before starting any treatment, you should also discuss with your dermatologist your medical history as well as any products you are using.

PRESCRIPTION-STRENGTH SKIN TREATMENTS

FREEZE

Botox

Botox Cosmetic is a nonsurgical treatment that works by blocking nerve impulses to the injected muscles. The prescription medication is injected into muscles to relax them and thus minimize the appearance of fine to deeper lines, most often around the eyes and on the forehead. Results are immediate and usually improve within days. The treatment lasts up to four months. Botox is also used to prevent wrinkling in areas that are dominated by deeper lines such as between brows. It is often used to lift fallen brows and eyes as well.

Xeomin

Xeomin is a prescription medication injected with a fine needle into wrinkle-causing muscles. It's similar to Dysport and Botox. Xeomin is often a matter of preference for the dermatologist and patient. It is often used to temporarily improve the look of moderate to severe frown lines and treat abnormal spasms of the eyelids and neck (Dystonia).

Dysport

Dysport, a purified protein, is injected using a fine needle, often to smooth out wrinkles. When performed correctly it can offer a more natural-looking result. It is effective in areas where overactive muscles cause frown lines and crease the skin. Dysport is similar to and used as an alternative to Botox; this is often a matter of preference for the dermatologist and the patient. Some doctors prefer Dysport when treating underarm sweat because it tends to spread to a wider area.

With botulinum toxin products Botox, Xeomin, and Dysport, side effects can range from discomfort in the injection site, blurred vision, and drooping eyelids or swelling of the eyelids to flulike symptoms; problems swallowing, speaking, or breathing; and (though rare) in severe cases, can result in death.

Fibro Cell Therapy

This is often used in lieu of Botox or Restylane. A dermatologist inserts your own cells, fibroblasts, which use your own skin tissue to add collagen back into your face. Tissue samples are removed from behind the ear and sent to the lab to multiply by the millions. Then they are injected back into the face to fill in smile lines and wrinkles around the lips. Unlike hyaluronic acid, the patient's own fibroblasts continue to work for years. The downside to this procedure is that it's time-consuming. The results are not immediate (you'll need three separate sessions) and treatments are expensive (around $5,000 each). Because it's a new procedure, there is still limited available data on the subject but fibro cell therapy is FDA approved and loved by many.

IPL (Intensive Pulsed Light)

IPL is often used to treat rosacea, sun damage, fine and large broken capillaries, and dark circles by instantly zapping away visible redness and stimulating collagen. The treatment feels a little like a rubber band being snapped lightly across the skin. Eyes are covered to protect them. A cooling gel is applied to the areas that are being treated. Targeted areas of the skin are stimulated using controlled application of broad spectrum high-intensity light.

The skin can remain pink for several days; other side effects include headaches and burning.

LIFT

This outpatient procedure can be performed by your dermatologist or a certified practitioner. It tightens and rebuilds the layers of the skin using radiofrequency or ultrasound technology. The choice is often what the practitioner is more comfortable using.

Thermage

A cooling agent is applied to the surface of the skin for protection, and gentle vibrations of radiofrequency are pointed into the skin using a tool. A cooling agent is then reapplied.

Using radiofrequency waves to penetrate all the layers of the skin helps rebuild collagen and tighten the skin. This is a great option if you are thinking of a face-lift, and is also great for handling contouring of the skin. Thermage is effective in tightening the jawline and lifting sagging cheeks as well as eyelids. Improvements continue for two to three months and last for up to six months.

Ulthera

This nonsurgical procedure stimulates the supporting layers of the skin. It uses ultrasound technology to heat the layers under the surface of the epidermis and uses your skin's own healing process to lift, tone, and tighten loose skin. Results happen in two to three months and continue for up to nine months. Procedures typically take sixty to ninety minutes.

VEINS

Compression Stockings

Compression stockings are the most natural way to reduce the risk of varicose veins as they promote circulation in the legs. They can be found online or at department stores and mass retailers. Compression stockings are a necessity for those who are sitting or standing for long periods of time. Remember, too, to put your legs above your heart for several minutes each day.

Ligation

Varicose veins can be surgically removed by a process called ligation and stripping. It is used on large, thick veins that often look blue and gray and are piling up in areas of the leg. The vein is removed by cutting at the top and bottom of the affected area and pulling the vein out. Since varicose veins are superficial veins, there is no real risk associated with the procedure.

Laser Ablation

Scelartherapy is a medical procedure performed to remove spider veins (little unsightly scatters of veins that occur in the legs) as well as varicose veins (large veins that can often look thick blue and gray and look like they are piling up in areas of the legs).

A microfoam is injected directly into the vein and is often less invasive, requiring less downtime. Remove any lotions prior to the procedure.

FILLERS

Young skin has a lot of hyaluronic acid, which the body naturally produces to bind water to the skin. As we age we produce less of this "youth serum," which results in less moisture and elasticity in the skin. Fillers are used to plump areas that have sunken or to give the illusion of fullness. Often, these fillers are used above the cheekbone and around the mouth in what are known as the "marionette lines," in the hollows of the cheeks, under the eyes, and to fill creases in the lip lines. Results are immediate, providing instant gratification.

Some doctors prefer to work with different fillers for different areas on the face, as the viscosity varies from product to product. There are several popular treatment options.

Restylane/ Juvéderm

Arguably one of the most popular injections to minimize the look of aging. These are both thick, gel-like substances that contain hyaluronic acid. These are often injected into marionette lines to fill in creases and to fill in cheeks.

Radiesse

This filler consists of calcium hydroxylapatite microspheres. It lasts up to twelve months, which is longer than Restylane or Juvéderm, but is more expensive. Radiesse is said to be a smoother compound than the others and contains a higher concentration of hyaluronic acid. It also contains a collagen builder and volumizing filler. Radiesse is often also used as a nose filler.

Sculptra

This filler uses poly-L-lactic acid to inject longer-lasting (up to two years) filler for areas with substantial loss of volume such as hollow cheeks. Sculptra is not suggested to fill in lines but rather to create fullness in the face that can be lost with age. It is injected into one of the lower layers of skin to promote collagen growth. Results do not happen immediately, but become visible within a few weeks. You may also need a few sessions for optimal results.

>>> Inside Secrets of a Dermatologist
Jessica Wu, MD

Dr. Jessica Wu is a cosmetic dermatologist practicing in Los Angeles. A graduate of Harvard Medical School, she is assistant clinical professor of dermatology at USC Medical School, and is involved in clinical research trials on injectable and topical antiaging treatments. Dr. Wu is a member of the Medical Nutrition Council of the American Society for Nutrition, and is author of *Feed Your Face: Younger, Smoother Skin and a Beautiful Body in 28 Delicious Days*. She shares some of the most common treatments for aging skin issues.

What Is the Best Treatment for Sagging Under the Eyes?

Sagging is usually caused by fat pockets or loose skin. If the cause is fat pockets, a lower-eye lift will tuck the fat pad back into place. If the issue is loose skin and fine lines under the eyes, it may improve with a TCA (trichloroacetic acid) chemical peel, which smooths and provides a little tightening as well.

Sagging may be exacerbated by fluid retention or inflammation (allergies, sinus problems) so anti-inflammatory products are often helpful. Eye creams with soy or green tea are natural anti-inflammatories. Avoid rubbing your eyes, especially late at night (so you don't wake up with puffy eyes). Cotton balls soaked in cold soymilk or green tea and applied to eyelids can help decrease puffiness.

HOW MANY TIMES BEFORE YOU SEE RESULTS?

One treatment for both eyes
TCA peel: $850
Upkeep
TCA peel: Once every year or two

What Is the Best Treatment for a Sagging Jawline?

ePrime is a radiofrequency treatment that uses a row of fine needles to deliver heat into the deeper layers of the skin. Clinical trials have shown results to be 35 percent as effective as a face-lift in sharpening the jawline and tightening looseness on the lower face. ePrime is a very popular procedure in my office and is safe for Asian, Hispanic, olive, and darker complexions, too, since it's not a laser treatment. The procedure takes about one and a half hours to perform, and is usually done under local anesthetic, so patients can drive themselves home. There will be seven to ten days of swelling and possible bruising. One treatment lasts, on average, for two years.

HOW MANY TIMES BEFORE YOU SEE RESULTS?

One time. Most patients see results within six to eight weeks, and continue to see improvement up to six months after their treatment.
Cost: $4,000
Upkeep: Every two years

IS THERE AN OVER-THE-COUNTER OPTION?

Algenist serum with alguronic acid, which has been shown to increase collagen and elastic tissue production. Elastic tissue helps keep your skin firm. Copper-containing creams are also good; copper is essential for making strong, elastic tissue.

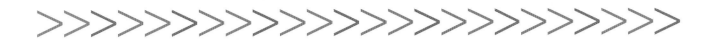

What Is the Best Treatment for Sagging Lids?

If sagging lids are caused by excess upper eyelid skin, then surgery to remove the excess skin is the best option. If the lids are slightly sagging, I often use a combination of Botox just under the tail of the eyebrow along with Juvéderm along the brow bone to lift the upper lid a few millimeters. This is often enough to open the eyes and make them look brighter and more awake. A new product, Neotensil, is a polymer film that temporarily tightens the under-eye area. It's a gel you apply in the morning, and it tightens as it hardens, lasting up to a day. It's only available in dermatologists' and plastic surgeons' offices.

HOW MANY TIMES BEFORE YOU SEE RESULTS?

One treatment for Botox/Juvéderm
Cost: $700 to $900 for Botox/Juvéderm
Upkeep: Every four to six months for Botox/Juvéderm

What Is the Best Treatment for Sagging Brows?

Botox can be used to lift the forehead and brow. (Xeomin or Dysport, which are newer alternatives to Botox, can also be used.) These treatments must be done by someone very experienced in doing injectables who can target the right muscles and maintain balance; otherwise you may get too much lift (and look shocked, or like Mr. Spock); or, you might end up with a heavier brow.

HOW MANY TIMES BEFORE YOU SEE RESULTS?

One treatment with Botox/Xeomin/Dysport
Cost: $450 to $800 for Botox/Xeomin/Dysport, depending on how many areas are treated. For some patients, I treat the frown and crow's-feet area as well, to maximize the lift and for a more natural look (otherwise your forehead may be smooth and lifted but your eyes will be wrinkled).
Upkeep: Every three to four months for Botox/Xeomin/Dysport

What's the Best Treatment for Marionette Lines?

Juvéderm or Restylane filler. Marionette lines are caused by thinning of the skin and loss of volume in the lower face, so it is also important to use over-the-counter products that contain vitamin C, an essential cofactor for building collagen.

HOW MANY TIMES BEFORE YOU SEE RESULTS?

Results are visible immediately, after just one treatment. The product tends to build over subsequent treatments, however, so the area looks better and better with each treatment and results last longer with further treatments.

Cost: $750 to $1,500 per treatment, depending on how much product is needed and how deep the lines are
Upkeep: Every 4 to 6 months initially, for the first two to three times, then every six to eight months

PLASTIC SURGERY

Technology has evolved so much with regard to skin treatment that plastic surgery can often be avoided. Taking care of yourself and getting noninvasive procedures done regularly can keep skin smooth and lifted, leaving surgery practically unnecessary. There are often circumstances, however, where surgery may be a practical option. Mastectomy, severe excess loose skin, or challenges after childbirth can make surgery preferable for some women to feel more secure with themselves. Brow lifts, eye surgery, and lower-face-lifts are often used to create longer-lasting effects. Going under the knife should be taken very seriously. If this is something you feel is right for you, it is essential to be educated and prepared. Do your research, make sure you're in optimum health, and exhaust other options first. When choosing a doctor, use the following checklist from the website of the American Society of Plastic Surgeons (plasticsurgery.org) as a guide during your consultation:

Are you certified by the American Board of Plastic Surgery?

Are you a member of the American Society of Plastic Surgeons?

Were you trained specifically in the field of plastic surgery?

How many years of plastic surgery training have you had?

Do you have hospital privileges to perform this procedure? If so, at which hospitals?

Is the office-based surgical facility accredited by a nationally- or state-recognized accrediting agency, or is it state-licensed or Medicare-certified?

How many procedures of this type have you performed?

Am I a good candidate for this procedure?

Where and how will you perform my procedure?

How long of a recovery period can I expect, and what kind of help will I need during my recovery?

What are the risks and complications associated with my procedure?

How are complications handled?

What are my options if I am dissatisfied with the outcome of my surgery?

Do you have before-and-after photos I can look at for each procedure and what results are reasonable for me?

In addition:

How should I prepare for my procedure?

Do you have photos of the procedure?

Do you recommend any alternative procedures?

Get costs in writing.

If possible, get a referral, but continue to ask questions. Do not rush to surgery. Look at all options.

SOLUTIONS TO COMMON SKIN CHALLENGES

Not everyone's skin dries out when they age. Some get severely oily or develop acne unexpectedly as hormones change. Menopause can force you to rethink your skincare and makeup regimens, an illness can change your skin drastically, and rosacea can flare. The following pages offer some solutions to these very common problems.

MENOPAUSE

Menopause is the end of ovulation and a woman's fertility. During this transition and period of very physical change, symptoms you may face include osteoporosis, stress, dry skin, sallow skin, night sweats, hot flashes, and tearing eyes. Drink plenty of water and minimize caffeine intake. Moisturize face and body regularly and use hydrating toners and serums—but avoid applying too close to the lash line to avoid eye stinging.

MAKEUP DURING HOT FLASHES

- Carry a fan to keep cool to prevent foundation from smearing.
- Consider stick or cream foundations, which can have a higher melting point.
- Apply water-resistant or mineral makeup or dual powder on top of water-resistant sunscreen immediately after application; this will hold color on to the skin better.
- Apply concealer or foundation on eyelids to hold eye shadow in place.
- Keep a portable fan nearby when applying makeup to keep you cool and dry.
- Keep blush to a minimum if you tend to flush.
- Use pomade or cream brow products for stay-put brows. Set with brow powder for more staying power.

TEARING EYES

- Wear waterproof or water-resistant mascaras and eyeliners.
- Keep rolled-up tissues in your purse for watering eyes. Do not use cotton swabs or cotton balls for sensitive eyes, which can leave lint residue. Hold tissue at the inner corners of your eyes to soak up tears before they can ruin your eye makeup.

- Exercise regularly to keep hormones and stress at bay. Strengthening exercises are essential for keeping bones strong.
- Consider meditation and deep-breathing exercises to oxygenate cells and create calm.
- Consume caffeine in the morning only as afternoon tea or coffee can affect proper sleep.
- Create a sleep routine. You need a minimum of seven hours for proper cell function.

ROSACEA

Rosacea is a very common skin condition that causes skin to turn red and for some creates sores that look similar to acne. It can be triggered by something as simple as spicy foods. As hormones change, rosacea can become an increasing problem. Use nonsensitizing products to minimize flare-ups. Wash with lukewarm water and use light exfoliants. Use sunscreen and pigmented powders to reduce redness. Talk to your dermatologist about Intensive Pulsed Light therapy (see page 17), as it may be a great solution to keep rosacea in check.

SENSITIVE SKIN

As we age, skin can become sensitive due to a multitude of factors, including the environment and sun damage. Sensitive skin can be really difficult to work with because it can be very prone to acne or dry patches. Many products cause you to break out in rashes easily or maybe your face turns red at even the lightest touch. You may be allergic to specific ingredients in certain products, so check with your dermatologist. Test newer products at the back of the jawline for sensitivity.

Wash cosmetic brushes often using a shampoo that you are not sensitive to, rinse thoroughly, and lay flat on a towel to dry. Change sponges and puffs frequently to avoid contaminating your skin. Many puffs and sponges can be washed and reused as well.

Use exfoliants that are fruit-enzyme based and contain less than 5 percent acidity. Avoid exfoliants that contain walnuts. Make sure to wear sunscreen; try physical barriers such as titanium dioxide and zinc oxide rather than chemical sunscreens, which can be more sensitizing. Avoid squeezing or scratching your face, as both can cause lasting hyperpigmentation on the skin.

Tweeze or thread (hair removal using threads to pull unwanted hairs) the face rather than waxing; you can take a pain reliever prior to service to minimize pain.

POST ILLNESS

Getting back to normal after illness or a lengthy hospital stay is important. While you may want to just go back to your routine, you likely need to make a few adjustments.

To minimize the effects of menopause, which can affect you both physically and mentally, consider having your hormone levels checked. Look into herbal remedies, bioidentical hormones, and hormone therapy, which can replace loss of your body's natural hormones. Talk to your doctor about different options, as there are benefits and disadvantages to taking hormones, including an increased risk of cancer.

Side effects from illness often include:

- Sallow skin
- Red, puffy skin around the eyes
- Hair loss
- Dry skin
- Loss of definition in features from brow and lash hair loss
- Hollow cheeks

First and foremost, keep products safe and bacteria-free. If you are still undergoing treatments or radiation, talk to your doctor, as even the smallest amount of bacteria can be a problem with a decreased immune system.

- Wash your hands thoroughly before touching your face.
- Use disposable mascara wands.
- Don't double-dip in products.
- Use a scraping tool with blushes and powders as well as eye shadows and lipsticks to get fresh product every time.
- Sharpen eye pencils (although pencils can be more difficult to adhere smoothly on textured skin).
- Use gel or cream eyeliners, as they glide better on textured skin after treatment.
- Clean brushes after every use.
- Never share products.
- Adding color is key to create the illusion of healthy skin (see page 48).
- Avoid cosmeceutical products and anything containing retinol or advertising keywords such as *antiaging*. Focus on products that are made for sensitive skin, and are labeled "hydrating."
- Use fluid foundation for healthy looking skin.
- Keep it simple.

Add Color to Lips

When circulation is poor, lips can turn a dull color and appear lifeless. Gently exfoliate the area using a warm washcloth then apply a heavy moisturizing balm. Apply lip liner to redraw the shape of lips, which can lose definition, and fill in using short strokes at the center of the mouth to blend color. Finish using a sheer or creamy lipstick to add color and moisture.

Fill in Brows

Lush eyebrows are a sign of health and vibrancy. To fill in sparse eyebrows, start with a lighter color first to create the outline of the brows. Fill in with the same color, using individual strokes to re-create lighter hairs. Then finish with a darker color to create darker strokes. This duplicates the look of natural eyebrows. If you have difficulty creating an outline, use stencils to help you create a guide then continue with individual strokes. Try pomades for dry skin, as pencils can often tug on dry skin and powders can sometimes be difficult to adhere.

Darken Foundation

During this time when you've likely been indoors due to illness or pale from loss of circulation, use a foundation one half to one full shade darker than your current skin tone to add color and even skin tone. Look for tinted or sheer foundation, as thinner skin can have difficulty carrying heavy foundation.

Stay away from powder or keep to a minimum as dry skin does absorb a lot of the moisture from foundations.

Freshen Cheeks

Illness can draw in cheeks and make them lose their vibrancy, creating a sallow, gaunt look. Add a natural rosiness and fullness to the face by simply applying a small amount of cream blush to the apple of the cheeks. Look for a color that your body naturally creates when flushed. For longer-lasting power, apply a powder blush on top in one shade lighter. Look for light shimmer to create the illusion of glowing cheeks. For the best results, smile to exaggerate apples of cheeks before applying.

ADULT ACNE

You probably thought worrying about acne was over after your teenage years were gone but acne occurs for many reasons: changes in hormone levels, stress, overuse of cosmetics, and changes in environment. I once gave advice to an eighty-year-old with chronic cystic acne. To treat acne, avoid touching your face. Keep pillows clean, and clean phones and anything else that might touch your face. Make sure to exfoliate skin as well as hydrate it, especially the areas that are prone to excess oil. Ask your dermatologist about a topical antibacterial or antibiotic treatment; your case may be slight enough that you simply need to change face-cleansing products, or you may need stronger medication. Give new products recommended to you a chance; many times you'll have initial breakouts because of the underlying clogged pores before skin starts to clear.

Don't forget that what you put in your body can affect your skin. Excessive amounts of caffeine can dehydrate skin. Skin works and looks its best when properly hydrated, so make sure to minimize the caffeine and drink plenty of hydrating fluids. Consider eating good fats such as avocado and fish, which can help minimize inflammation in the skin.

For heavy acne, apply mineral or dual foundation powder and apply spot concealer on any remaining discoloration from blemishes afterward to minimize the appearance of caking.

Look for sunscreens that are zinc or titanium dioxide based; these physical sunscreens are less oily than chemical sunscreens.

DRY SKIN

As we age, oil glands slow production and we lose hyaluronic acid in our skin, which once helped us retain up to one thousand times its weight in water.

Use hydrating toners prior to serums and moisturizers to help normalize the skin. They also help the skin to better absorb the ingredients. Use liquid exfoliants/toners containing alpha hydroxy acids such as glycolic acid or retinoids to remove dead skin cells, which can accumulate on the surface. Make sure to use serums with peptides and hyaluronic acid to deliver and trap more moisture in the skin. Avoid hot showers to prevent overdrying. Make sure to use separate eye cream for the delicate eye area. Chemical sunscreens can be less drying if titanium dioxide or zinc oxide is a problem for your skin.

Applying makeup to seriously dry skin is easier using creamier products. Cream blushes can add luminosity to skin, and cream liners glide on smoothly as pencils can tug and give an uneven application. Powder for setting foundation may not be necessary if your skin is absorbing the oils from the foundation. To set, try using a very small amount of loose powder, which will not have the extra ingredients such as binding agents that pressed powders do.

MATURING OILY SKIN

Not all maturing women have dry skin. Often, women who have thicker and naturally oily skin can have less fine lines as they age but can also have enlarged pores and very active sebaceous glands. While the oily skin can be protecting the outer layer of the skin, the underlying layers are still going through the motions of collagen loss, especially if not taken care of properly. Avoid using washcloths or abrasive scrubs, which can scratch the surface and cause inflammation and damage to delicate skin. Use mattifying skin primers on areas with excess oil after applying moisturizer, and before sunscreen, and foundation.

Foundation

Use an oil-free foundation to even out skin tone if necessary. I personally prefer using stick or cake foundations on oily areas because they offer so much pigment in a little amount of product and can feel lighter to the skin. Be sure to blend well so that the product is in a thin layer and doesn't cake.

Concealers

Use cake or stick concealers, as they'll hold on to oily areas better than liquid concealers. For the under-eye area, which can have a different texture, use liquid, cream, or stick concealers.

BLACKHEADS

Use a clay mask once a week to remove blackheads and other impurities in the skin. Make sure to wear moisturizers to regulate oil production, as excess oil is often a sign that your body is trying to make up for skin's lack of moisture. Use products containing acids and retinoids to minimize large pores, and make sure to cleanse thoroughly twice a day, as oils can also attract dust and dirt. Wear physical sunscreens that contain titanium dioxide or micronized zinc oxide, which are less greasy than chemical sunscreens. Avoid squeezing blackheads as the pressure can cause damage to the skin and create hyperpigmentation.

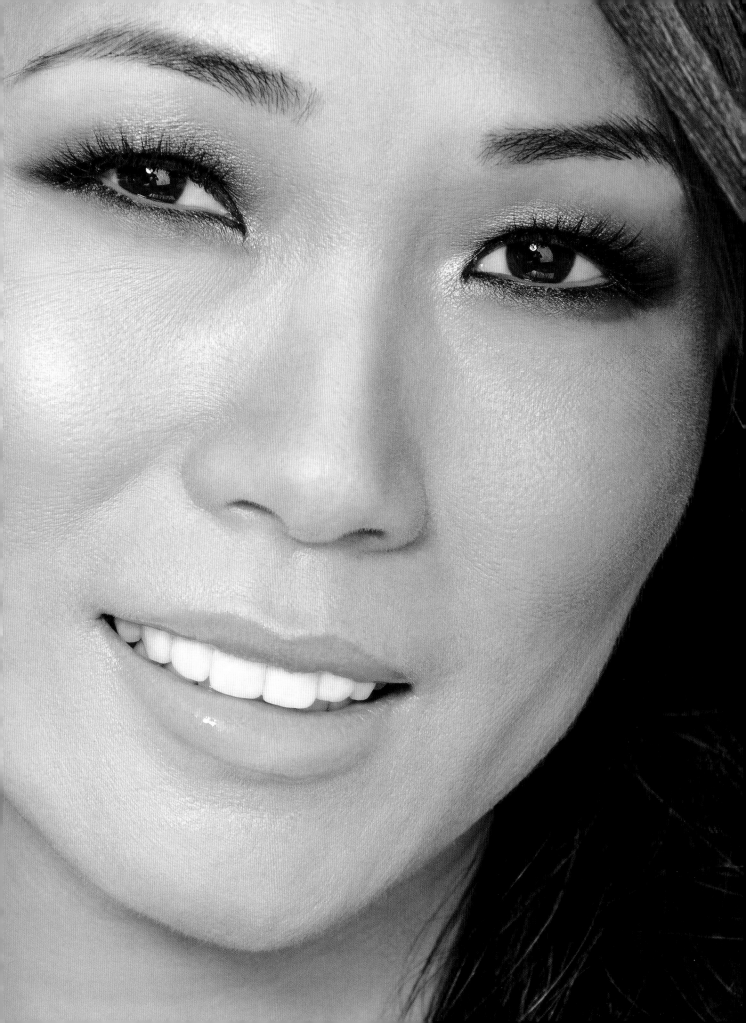

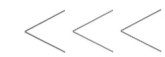

FOUNDATION

Creating Flawless Second Skin

Proper foundation and concealer application will create the illusion of flawless, more youthful skin. The right foundation should blend in with your skin and make you appear fresh and healthy. It should never appear caked on. Proper foundation doesn't compete with sunspots or uneven skin tone; it simply puts the focus back on your most beautiful facial features and gives you younger-looking skin.

CHOOSING FOUNDATION

You've heard of all the bizarre places to test foundation like the inside of your wrist, but the best place to test your color is on your jawline. This way your foundation will blend with your neck and there will be no line of demarcation, or what I call "a floating face." When choosing foundations, consider undertone, texture, and shade.

If you have very uneven skin tone (for instance, a dark forehead and a lighter jawline) or full-faced freckles, choose a foundation color in between your two shades. You can also contour (see contouring section page 47).

UNDERTONE

It's important to find out which undertone your skin has. Cool skin has a pink undertone, warm skin has a bronze undertone, and neutral skin has a yellow undertone. You can see the tones easier when you lay several colors in the same shade next to each other. This makes the difference in colors stand out more. To see which undertone is closest to you, place on your jawline.

Choose a few different foundations that seem closest to your skin tone and apply vertically on the jawline so that you can see at least an inch of each color. Look in the mirror about a foot away from your face so that you can see the overall picture. The foundation you choose should appear invisible because it blends so well into your skin.

Note: Dark skin will often have warm undertones on the forehead with more neutral, golden undertones in the under-eye area and may require you to purchase two different shades for the best application.

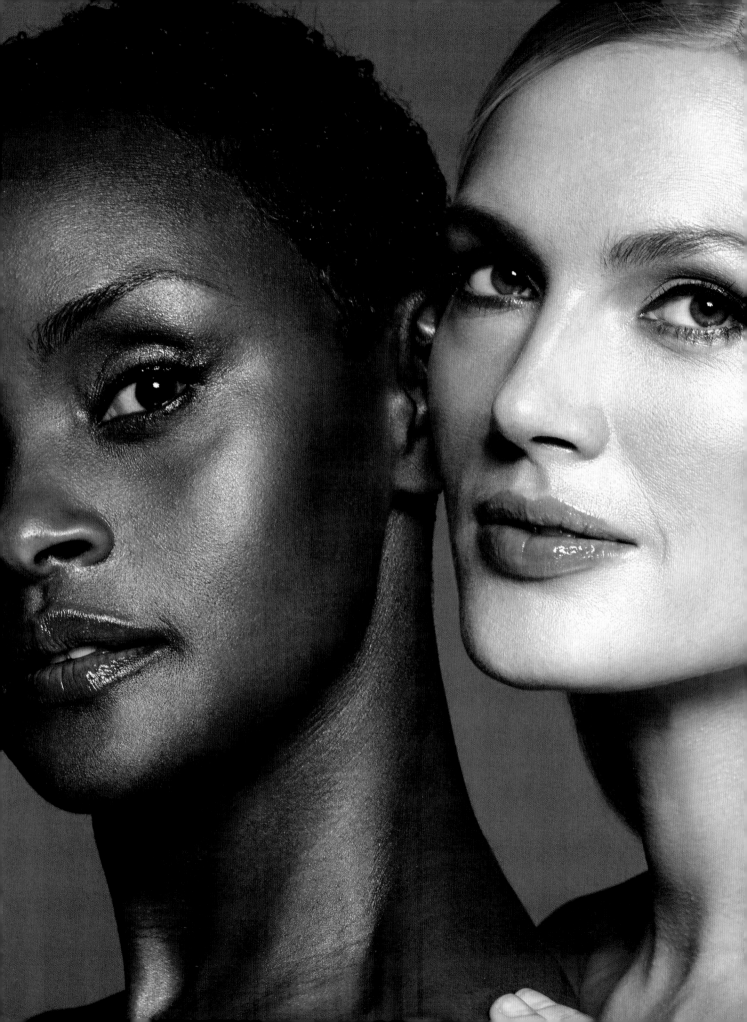

TEXTURE

Lighter Coverage

Lighter-coverage foundation that is mostly clear is a perfect option for mature skin that just needs a little color to even out skin tone. These are also easy and fast to apply, which is perfect for those of us without a lot of time for a complicated morning makeup routine.

TINTED MOISTURIZER

This is the sheerest of bases, offering a hint of color added to moisturizer; most varieties contain sunscreen as well. Most come in yellow-based tones and they are so sheer that they blend into most skin tones.

BB CREAM

Standing for beauty balm or blemish balm, BB cream is an all-purpose foundation that promises to replace moisturizer, foundation, and sunscreen. It offers sheer to medium coverage.

SHEER FOUNDATION

The lightest in texture of the foundation family, this is great for women who still have excellent skin tone and don't want too much coverage. I prefer water-/silicone-based foundations as they mix well with most moisturizers and work well with dry to oily skin.

FLUID FOUNDATION

This type of foundation is generally found in a bottle. It comes in a variety of textures including very sheer, but can also contain more pigment and provide medium coverage.

Medium Coverage

CREAM FOUNDATION

Available in pots or tubes these medium- to full-coverage foundations contain more pigment, which creates a thicker consistency. They are great for combination skin as they work well on oily as well as dry areas. Apply lightly on areas that require less coverage and more heavily on discolored skin such as the cheek area, which can have more skin damage like rosacea or hyperpigmentation, and the nose area, which can have broken capillaries and redness.

MINERAL POWDER

Loose minerals are used in place of foundation to deliver sheer to medium coverage (depending on the amount applied). While offering a slight shimmer to re-create glow in dulling skin, powder does lack the suppleness that fluid foundations can create. It is a great alternative, however, for those with thick, deep wrinkles where foundation can settle and crease, or for people in hot, humid climates. After applying, try lightly spraying the face with aerosol water vapors to set the powder into the skin and create more glow.

Full Coverage

CAKE FOUNDATION

Found in compact or stick form, these give the most amount of coverage because they contain very dense pigment; this also makes the formula drier than other foundations. I prefer cake foundation for skin that requires very full coverage, as well as oily skin. Because of cake foundation's consistency and dense pigment, you can use very little for less coverage and it is less likely to slide or melt off oily skin. It is also great for humid climates or during menopause, when moisture during hot flashes can cause makeup to slide (it has a higher melting point than fluid foundations).

FOUNDATION POWDER

A heavily pigmented powder can be used on top of foundation to give heavy-duty coverage or in place of foundation. This works best on skin with heavy acne or thick wrinkles, and is also great for humid climates. Apply using a large powder brush for sheer coverage or a powder puff for full coverage.

SHADE

Once you've found your favorite foundation and appropriate color, it's best to also buy an additional one in one shade lighter or darker than your usual color. Most skin colors do change half to one shade throughout the year depending on the season. If you're using the lighter foundation shade (usually during winter), use the darker under the cheekbones to define them. If you're using your darker shade (for summer), use the lighter foundation along the middle of your nose and under eyes as a highlighter. If you forget which foundation to use, just remember that dark shades make features recede and light shades make features more prominent.

To neutralize pink skin, apply a yellow-based foundation to cancel out any discoloration in the cheeks and visible capillaries that can occur with aging, thinning skin or rosacea.

TOOLS

SPONGE

Sponges release less product than other application tools, making them excellent for blending. You can also use sponges to blend out foundation if you've applied too much using the other tools. Sponges absorb almost twice as much product, however, so you are likely to go through your foundation faster. Use disposable sponges for sensitive skin to reduce possible irritation from leftover product; if you have an expensive reusable sponge, wash regularly using mild soap and warm water. For more sheer coverage, apply foundation using a wet sponge. Tap foundation using sponges onto areas needing extra coverage due to skin discoloration or hyperpigmentation.

Allow moisturizer to settle into skin for a few moments before applying any foundation; this ensures a better blend.

FINGERS

The heat of your fingers warms foundation and can help to better blend it into the skin. They are nature's tool to get into smaller areas of the face. Use ring and middle finger to apply a gentler application of foundation applying downward with the growth of the hair. Use your ring finger (this will give you the lightest touch) to tap on concealer or a second layer of foundation on areas that might need it. Make sure your hands are clean and apply foundation using small quantities at a time. If you've just gotten a manicure you may want to opt for using a different tool as foundation can get stuck under fingernails.

FOUNDATION BRUSH

Usually made of synthetic fibers (which absorb less product) a foundation brush gives the best application control, doesn't suck up a lot of product, and keeps your fingers clean. Apply downward with growth of hairs. Choose a brush that thins out at the tip to help blend and tap on additional layers on areas of the face that might need it. I prefer synthetic fibers made of high-quality taklon. Wash according to manufacturer's instructions—usually shampoo and warm water at least once a week and lay flat to dry.

THE PROPER AMOUNT

FOREHEAD

While the forehead is a larger area of the face, it actually requires less foundation as it tends to have thinner skin and deeper lines. Use a lighter amount of foundation and/or powder, as a heavier application can exaggerate lines.

EYELIDS

The skin on the lids is very thin compared to the rest of the face, which causes veins and discoloration to appear more visible. Foundation on the eyelids not only helps eye shadow stay on longer, it hides any discoloration of the skin. Start from the inner corners of the lids and move gently to the outer corners.

CHEEKS

The cheek area requires the most amount of foundation as it is the largest surface area of the face and usually holds a lot of discoloration, whether from age spots, hyperpigmentation, or rosacea. Start with the most foundation at the apples of the cheek and move out and downward.

NOSE

Apply foundation along the sides and below the nose onto the upper lip to hide melasma (patches of dark skin) or broken capillaries around the nose. Tap on additional foundation if necessary to fill in large pores.

CHIN

Apply a small amount of foundation to the chin area and work up into the lower lips and under the jawline.

NECK

Make sure to blend foundation into the jaw and neckline so that there is no line of demarcation.

APPLICATION

Before applying foundation you should always prep your face by washing, exfoliating, and moisturizing your skin. This ensures the smoothest base for foundation and results in the most even and natural-looking foundation application.

Be sure to test primer with your current foundation. Primers have different functions: to fill large pores, smooth fine lines, mattify oily skin, or simply allow a smoother application of foundation. The wrong primer, on the other hand, can leave foundation looking separated or pasty. Consider using primer made specifically for your particular foundation; many companies offer companion products. Allow primer time to dry before applying foundation.

Applying foundation downward, in the same direction that your hairs grow, creates the most natural application and makes facial hairs less visible. Refer to the previous sections to choose appropriate tools and the correct amount of foundation to apply to each part of the face.

For thick, deep wrinkles, avoid large amounts of foundation; instead, try pigmented powder and spot-apply concealer on top of powder where necessary.

Your foundation should evolve with your skin, so change products as necessary. As you get older skin gets thinner and discolorations can become more visible. The body also creates less melanin, so skin loses color and can appear sallow. If your skin tone is uneven opt for foundation in a slightly darker shade. If broken capillaries or veins become more evident, switch to products that provide heavier coverage.

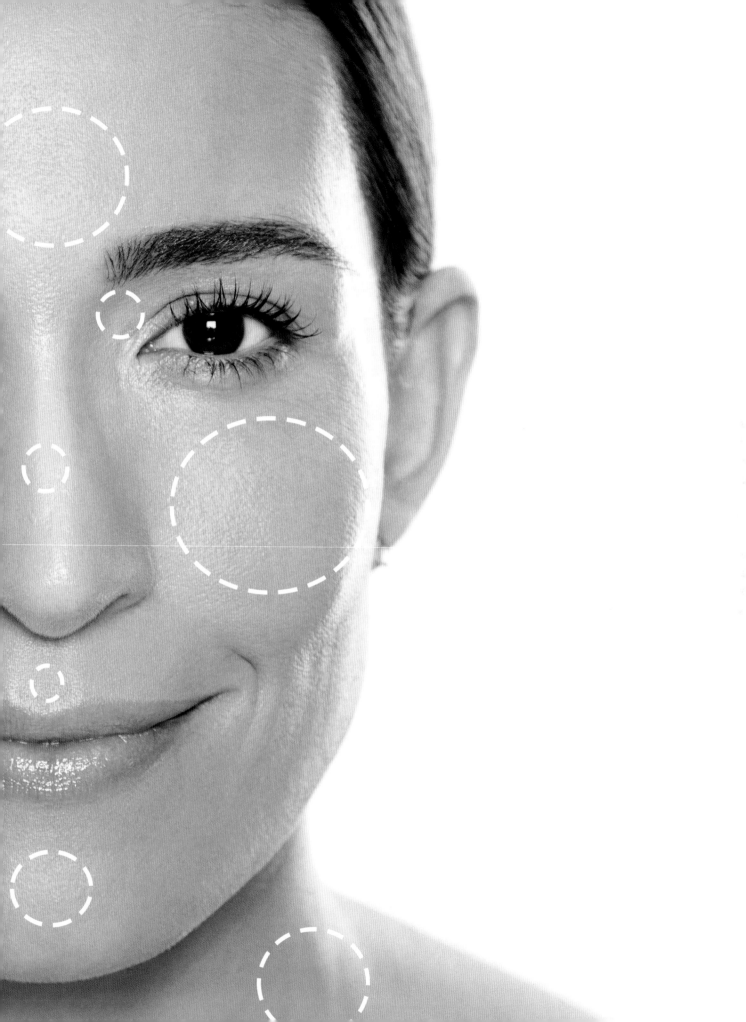

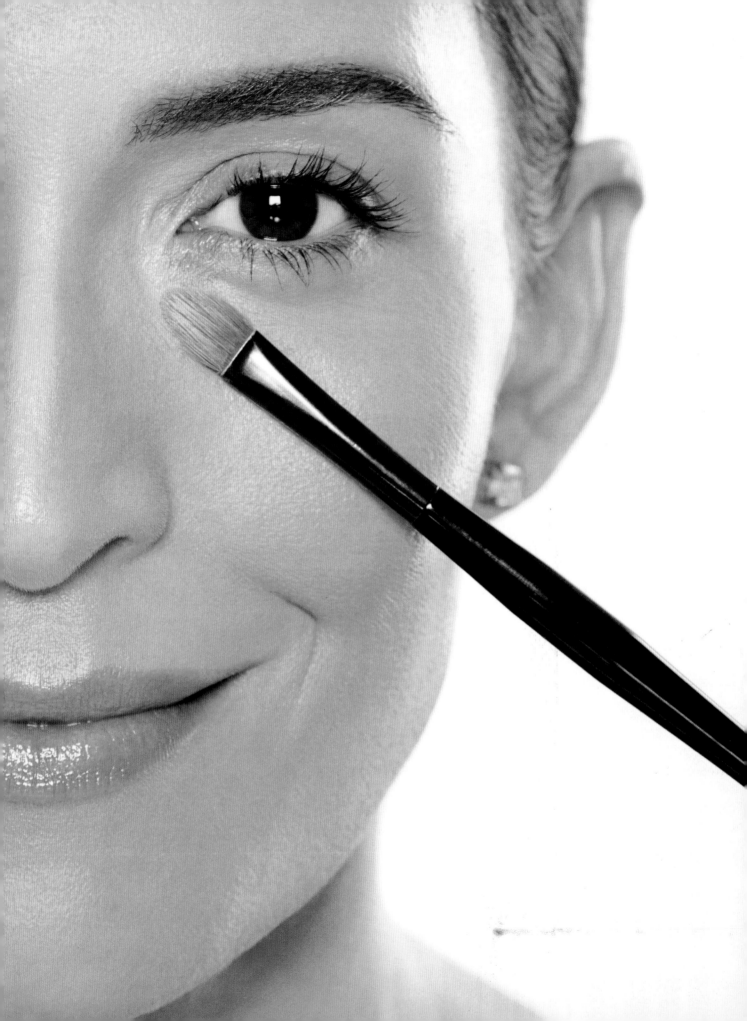

THE PERFECT CONCEALER

How to Apply and Choose Shades

As we age, many of us discover that the area around and under our eyes tends to become discolored with fine lines. The perfect concealer can change the eyes completely by hiding discoloration and brightening the area, giving the illusion of livelier, youthful eyes. On the skin, the right color also cancels out dark spots and blemishes. Make sure that you consider textures as well; the area under your eyes will be a different texture than the skin around your cheeks and product will set differently in different areas. And finally, it is essential to blend concealer into the skin to avoid any visible edges.

MINIMIZE CROW'S-FEET USING CONCEALER

Fine lines and wrinkles create darkness in the outer corners of the eyes. The lines cast shadow, which makes them even more apparent. Applying a concealer at an upward angle after all makeup is applied gives the illusion of lift to the eyes. Use a concealer brush and wipe across corners at a 45-degree upward angle to clean up any eyeliner errors and erase fine lines. Use a thin layer of cream or pen concealer, as it is less likely to settle into fine lines.

If under-eye makeup starts to settle into any fine lines, gently tap the area back and forth with your ring finger, using your finger's natural heat to blend makeup back into skin.

HOW TO APPLY CONCEALER

Apply foundation to even out skin first, and then tap on concealer to cover any remaining discoloration. This ensures you use the smallest amount of concealer possible. Applying concealer on top of foundation creates controlled coverage and minimal smearing.

TOOLS

Small synthetic concealer brushes provide precise coverage to hard-to-reach areas of the eyes like the inner corners, especially if you have deep-set eyes. The natural heat of fingers softens the concealer, however, and makes it easier to blend. Concealers for both under the eyes and on the face should be applied after foundation and before powder.

CHOOSING A TEXTURE

If your skin texture varies greatly it may be necessary to use different types of concealers: one in a thinner texture to highlight underneath the eyes, where the skin can often be thin, crepe-like, and dry; and the other for the face, where the texture is thicker and often requires heavier coverage in a cake or stick form. Use in a slightly darker shade than the under-eyes to conceal sunspots or any other imperfections.

CHOOSING A CONCEALER SHADE

When choosing the color of your concealer, avoid colors that are too light, which can look unnatural. Often when applying concealer, women make the mistake of thinking that dark circles under the eyes should be covered with the lightest concealer color possible, which can result in a light grayish halo under the eyes. Look for a concealer only a half shade to a full shade lighter than the skin color directly beneath your eyes and use undertones to cancel out darkness. The same applies to blemishes on the skin. If the imperfection is pink or red in color (such as a pimple or broken capillaries), choose a concealer with a yellow undertone. The yellow will cancel out the redness. If it's brown or black (such as a mole), choose one with a pink undertone; if it's blue (such as under-eye skin), choose one with slight orange or peach undertones.

Identifying Undertone

To identify what undertone a concealer contains, try laying out several swabs of different concealers side by side. The differences in undertones will appear more obvious when next to each other. Names can give a little away. Generally, ivory is light with a hint of pink; beige has a hint of peach; and ocher has a yellow undertone.

Concealer Product

PEN: These concealers are very light in texture but can cover light to medium imperfections. They're usually best used for fine lines under the eyes or if you have problems with creping (rough, dry texture, which causes the cosmetic to sit in the lines).

CREAM: Usually found in a tube, this texture is great for under the eyes as it contains more moisture while still delivering medium to heavy coverage. It's ideal for camouflaging dark circles.

STICK: This is a medium- to heavy-coverage concealer with similar texture to a cake but in stick form, and is usually less dense. Powdering after application is generally unnecessary as stick concealer stays in place on its own. Stick concealer works well for thicker skin, warm weather, or if you have problems with concealers staying on (good for women experiencing menopause).

CAKE: Very dense in texture and opaque in coverage, cake concealer usually delivers the most amount of pigment. It is commonly found in pot form. Cake concealer is great for areas or imperfections that require heavy coverage such as moles, dark spots, or tattoos. It's also ideal for oily skin or to cover scarring or bruising. For dry skin that needs heavy coverage, moisturize the area heavily prior to application. Avoid powdering after applying concealer for a more natural look. If you need to set it, apply a sheer layer of translucent powder.

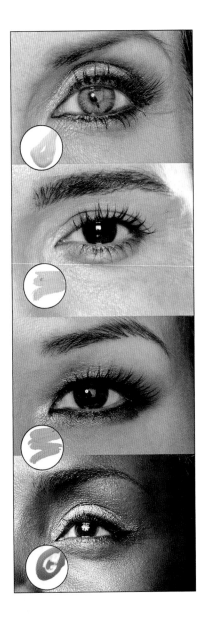

FAIR
For very pale skin, use concealers that have a slight yellow undertone, as skin can be thin and have a pink or purple hue under the inner corner of the eye.

MEDIUM
For medium skin tones, look for concealers in beige.

OLIVE
For olive skin tones, look for concealers in colors like ocher.

CARAMEL
For caramel skin tones, look for concealers in colors like golden honey.

DARK
Dark skin often needs concealer with more orange or slightly red undertones, as darkness will generally appear as deeper shades of the natural skin tone. This makes pink an ineffective concealer color. Look for the lightest color on your face and find a heavy cream or stick concealer one half and up to two shades lighter. For dark skin, look for concealers in colors like caramel or almond. You can also go as light as honey to add dramatic highlighting and create dimension in the skin.

COVERING BRUISES

It's inevitable; we are much more susceptible to bruising as we age. Thinning skin and aging capillaries that rupture and leak under the skin make the bruise more visible. A significant number of bruises occur at the injection sites for various beauty treatments. Make sure to tell your dermatologist if you are taking any prescription medications such as blood thinners or aspirin before any injections. I can't tell you how many women I've met who hide their treatments from their friends, coworkers, and even husbands. I suppose there is a certain amount of vanity that is exposed when others find out you've received a treatment, so to keep them guessing a little longer about how you stay so young, here's how to hide injection-site bruises if and when they come up (and any time they occur in general).

Apply foundation to the entire area using the lightest-texture product. This helps the area appear more blended with the face. Apply concealer to the bruised area using a small concealer brush or clean lip brush, making sure to tap the color on gently, and then blend out the outer edges into the rest of the skin. Set with translucent loose powder by gently brushing it onto the area, preferably using a small contour brush. Use a powder light in texture and sheer in color; pigmented powder can darken and draw more attention to the bruise.

Look for concealer a half shade to one full shade lighter than the surrounding area of the bruise and with the following cancelling undertones:

BRUISE COLOR	CONCEALER COLOR
Red	Yellow
Purple	Yellow-green
Blue	Orange
Green	Pink or orange
Yellow	Beigy-Pink
Black	Pink
Brown	Salmon or peach

Your foundation color - ½ to 1 shade + cancelling color = covered bruise

---

COVERING SPOTS AND MOLES

Moles and spots are generally black or brown and should not be covered simply by a lighter concealer, which can make the imperfection appear gray. Black moles should be covered by concealers with slightly pink undertones to cancel out the color, and brown spots can be cancelled out by slightly peach or salmon undertones. Try both to see which is right for you.

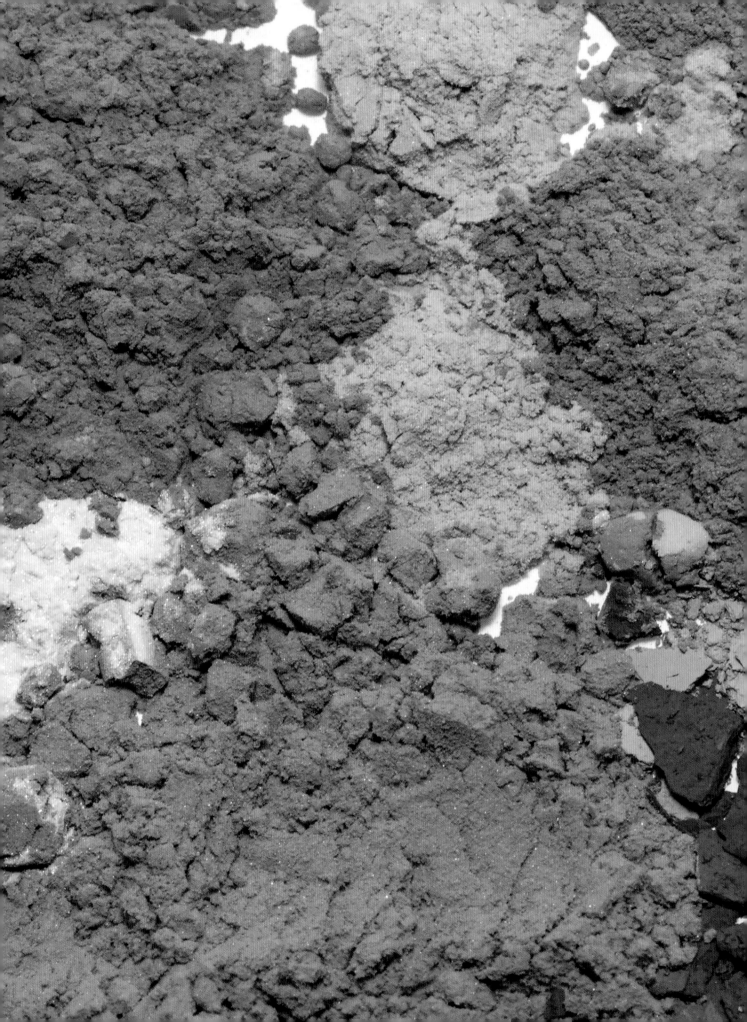

SETTING
FOUNDATION

Appropriate powder application is where many women go wrong. Even with the perfect foundation application, the wrong powder and tool can make skin appear a decade older. Setting foundation with powder keeps the makeup in place. Without this step, the heat of your body is certainly going to cause your foundation to rub off or run. Setting foundation can sometimes be an unnecessary step for women with extra dry skin; however, the emollients in the makeup are absorbed by dehydrated skin and can leave even fluid foundation semimatte, requiring little to no setting powder. If necessary, use a finely milled loose powder that contains a slight shimmer to add vibrancy and give the illusion of luminous, healthy skin.

As a general rule the heavier the foundation, the lighter the powder needs to be.

POWDER TYPES

Powders come in a wide variety of colors and textures, from sheer to opaque, and are easy to apply. They often contain oils and binding agents to hold their shape—a must for when you're on the go and need to prevent spills and messes. Apply with a large powder brush to get the most natural application.

SHEER PRESSED POWDER

Translucent powder in a pressed form is great for application on the go. It's a must to simply set foundation without additional bulk. Pressed powder is great for most skin types, but it's especially perfect for a natural finish on dry skin.

DUAL POWDER

Dual powder is a full-coverage pressed powder that can be used instead of foundation and provides an extra-matte finish. Choose a powder that's a half to a full shade darker than your skin tone to avoid appearing pasty. When using in conjunction with foundation for extra-heavy on-camera type coverage, its best applied with a powder brush to avoid a thick application. This is a great product for maturing, oily skin.

LOOSE POWDER

Loose powders set makeup while still maintaining skin's youthful finish. It is essential especially if you're using heavy foundation. Loose powder can be found in a variety of colors and because of its sheer texture, colors can be easily matched to your skin tone. They are also available in higher pigment formulas, which give more coverage but don't contain a lot of the extras like oils that are necessary to keep the powder in a pressed form. Loose powder is perfect for dry skin, as using it sets the foundation while maintaining the skins luminosity.

MINERAL POWDER

Used often in lieu of foundation, mineral powder contains mineral oxides and often has a slight shimmer, and provides light to medium coverage. Make sure to moisturize well prior to application and apply concealer after powder if necessary. Mineral powder is great for those who want light coverage and a matte finish. Best on skin with deep wrinkles and fairly even skin tone.

TRANSLUCENT POWDER

Available in loose and pressed form, a true translucent powder has no color and creates the sheerest setting of foundation. It's great for all skin types (but especially good for dry skin), to help set foundation. Choose powders that are finely milled and preferably in loose form to offer the lightest weight. Translucent powder can appear gray on darker skin; opt instead for powder with yellow or slightly orange undertones.

Oily Skin

Look for powders that contain silica to absorb excess oil. Blotting papers are a great option for aging, oily skin for touch-ups as they soak up oil without having to add additional powder which, at the end of the day, can appear cakey.

Dark Skin

Dark skin may require two different colors to set foundation. The forehead tends to be a lot darker than under the eyes or above the apples of the cheeks, and the forehead may have a red undertone where the apples may have a yellow undertone.

TOOLS

BRUSH

Use a soft, rounded powder brush to give you the most controlled application. Brushes deposit a small amount of powder with the least amount of absorption. Choose a large powder brush that tapers at the edges and is made of high-quality bristles. The hairs should be soft to the touch and made of taklon, goat, squirrel, or sable. Avoid hard-edged bristles and rough brushes. Not only can these irritate delicate skin, they will deposit powder unevenly.

To apply, use your brush to pick up powder and shake off any excess by lightly tapping the ferrule (strip closest to the bristles). Using a light touch, apply powder moving downward along the growth of facial hairs. The result is a smooth application of powder that blends into the skin.

POWDER PUFF

Puffs deposit the most amount of product because they make it easier to push it into the skin. To get a lighter application of powder using a puff, pick up powder with the puff and rub off any excess on the back of your hand or paper towel. Picking up small amounts allows you to control the volume of powder you use. Press the puff gently onto the skin in a rocking motion. Puffs are great for travel, if you have to touch up at work, or during a night out on the town.

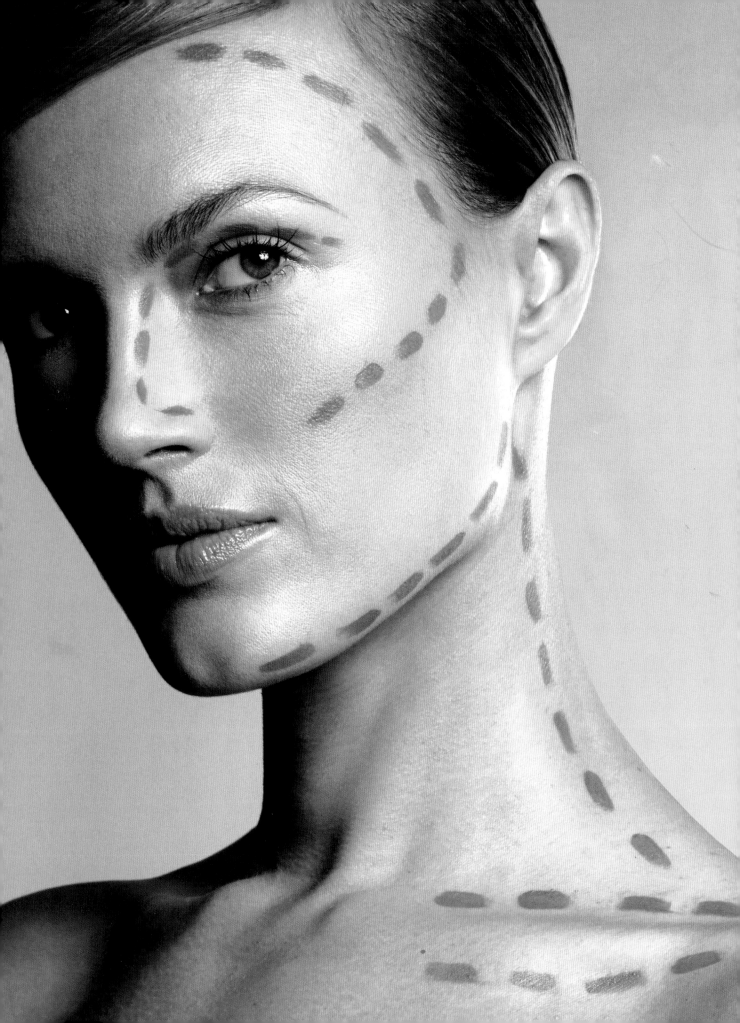

THE COLOR FACE-LIFT

Creating the illusion of an instant face-lift simply by using a few shades of foundation or bronzer to contour and highlight may seem like a stretch, but is surprisingly effective. When skin ages it loses color and becomes sallow, making sagging skin and its falling shadows appear more prominent. Contouring using foundation is simply redirecting the shadows to work in your favor. Use darker shades of foundation or bronzer to lift falling cheeks, minimize a sagging jawline, and add color to dull skin. Use highlight to bring forward sunken under-eyes, highlight the bridge of the nose, and lift brows.

CONTOURING

Contouring is basically redefining the edges of your features to create shape, using darker shades of foundation, powder, or bronzer. While this can be an intimidating concept for many women (possibly too many striped noses or sharp cheekbones in media have deterred many of us from trying this seemingly complex technique), when executed well, contouring actually re-creates the healthy, sun-kissed glow that can be lost as the skin becomes sallow during the aging process. It also helps to minimize the contrast between facial coloring and coloring on the chest or arms, which can often become more pronounced as we age.

CHOOSING A SHADE
Look to the natural skin tones on your body and choose the darkest shade. You'll notice that your chest or shoulders, and maybe even your forearms, are significantly darker than your face. Choosing a color your body naturally produces creates the

most natural look. Use foundations that are two or three shades darker than your natural skin tone for an even, more natural look.

Pale Skin

Stick with a soft, sheer light tawny brown one to two shades darker than your natural skin tone. Avoid any colors that have too much shimmer or have an orange undertone.

Very Dark Skin

Use your natural coloring as the contour color and reshape by highlighting the inside of your face (that is, under the eyes, the bridge of your nose, and your chin). Many women with dark skin have varying skin tones throughout the face—a natural contouring, you might say. When applying only one shade to the entire face you may find that the color makes you either appear too dark or ashy. This is because many times your forehead might be dark with red undertones while your T-zone area will be several shades lighter with yellow undertones. To get the best result, choose a foundation color closest to your forehead shade. Then choose a second color closest to the lightest shade on your face, which is generally under the eyes. You may also need two different setting powders, but the result will be a beautiful, perfect match.

ADDING COLOR

You can add more color and contour to the face by strategically applying bronzers and blushes. Apply contour shade from the temple along the underside of the cheekbone. Apply blush to the apples of the cheeks to create the illusion of fullness.

Apply bronzer contour color on the outside of the face and highlight colors in the center of the face. If the skin on your chest is darker, don't mix the colors along your neck; use your chest as the guide for the contour color.

It's important to keep the highlight and contour colors only a shade or two apart. This creates the most natural look and is also forgiving of mistakes. Blending and placement of shades is key with contouring. The center of the face (under the eyes and on the bridge of nose, bottom of the forehead, and chin) should always be lighter than the outer edges to highlight your features. It's important to blend the two lightly together so there are no harsh lines, but don't mix them completely. Rather, make sure to blend only the outer edges to gently connect the two colors together. An easy way to do this is to lightly brush the area where the contoured and non-contoured areas meet with a clean brush.

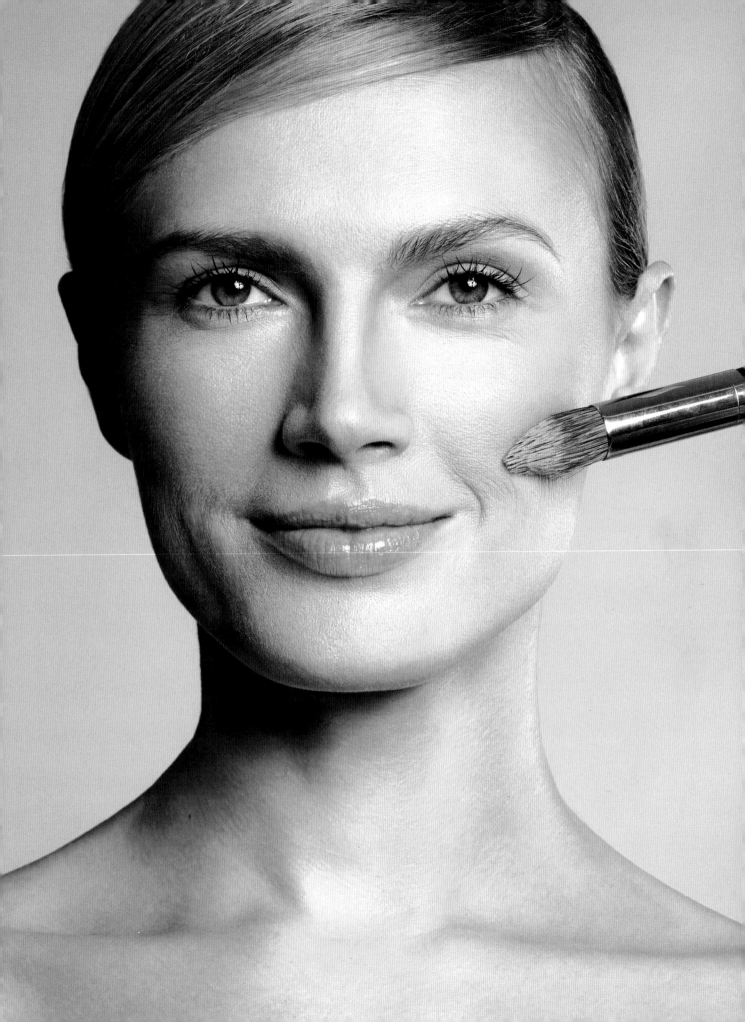

NATURAL FACE-LIFT

HIDING A THINNING HAIRLINE

Use a contour shade along the temples and hairline to minimize the forehead, which can appear larger due to a thinning hairline. Work color close into hairline so that there is no line of demarcation. This also creates a sun-kissed look.

CONTOURING MATURE SKIN

Apply contour shade from under the cheekbone toward the nose and blend up. This will create the illusion of lift for falling cheeks. For a wider face, move contour closer to the nose; for a narrow face, blend contour under the apples of the cheeks.

THINNING A WIDE NOSE

Our noses continue to grow as we age and can appear wider than we remember. Apply contouring shades along the sides of the nose from the inside of brows down to the tip of the nose and blend down the sides. Apply a straight line of highlighter along the bridge of the nose. The wider the highlighted area, the wider the nose will appear. The thinner the highlight, the thinner the nose.

Shadow the sides of the ball of the nose as well, to continue the illusion of a thinner nose. For a long tip of the nose, slightly shadow the underside of the nose to give the illusion of shorter length.

HIDING AN IMPERFECT NECKLINE

Apply a darker contour shade under the jawline and blend down into the neck area to create shadow. Make sure that the neck is moisturized well to ensure easier blending.

DEFINING THE COLLAR BONE

Apply darker contour shade along the top and bottom of the collarbones to create definition. For overly pronounced collarbones apply foundation over the entire collarbone area.

CREATING DEPTH IN EYES

Apply contour shade at the base of the lids to create depth, but be sure to avoid the brow bone. The shade should be applied higher than the natural crease of the eye to create the illusion of lift. Apply a highlighter shade under the arch of the brow to create lift.

Note: A natural contoured look can be achieved using foundation in different forms from sheer to stick foundations. The heavier the texture and darker the foundation, the stronger the contoured effect will be.

You can also achieve a bronzed effect with the use of bronzing powders in addition to foundation.

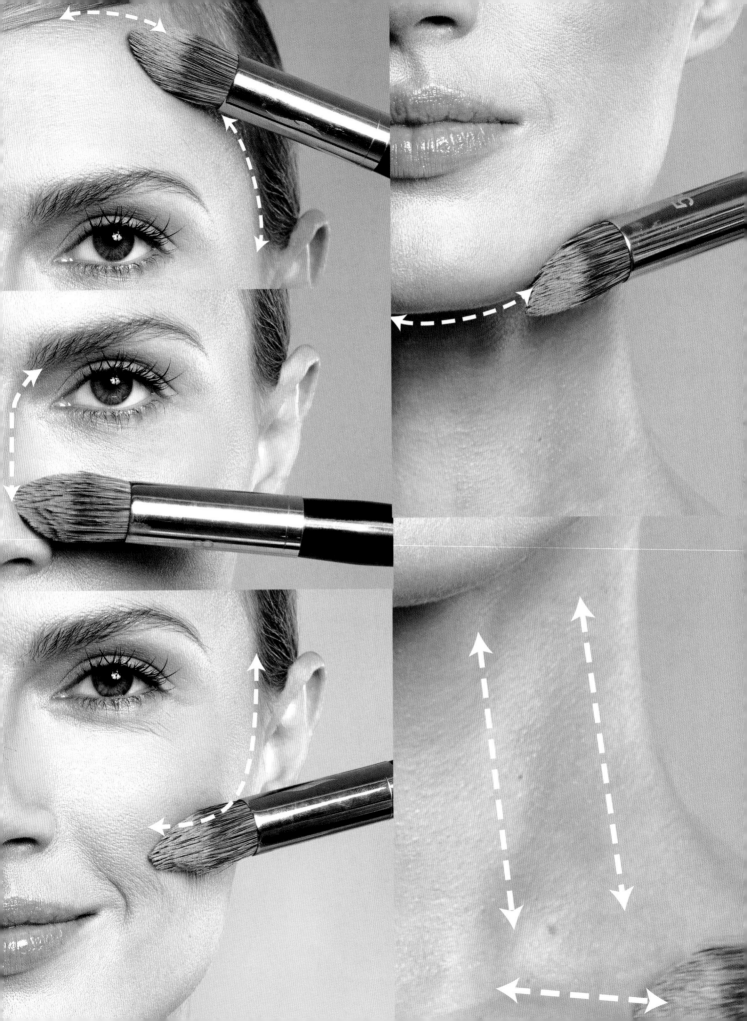

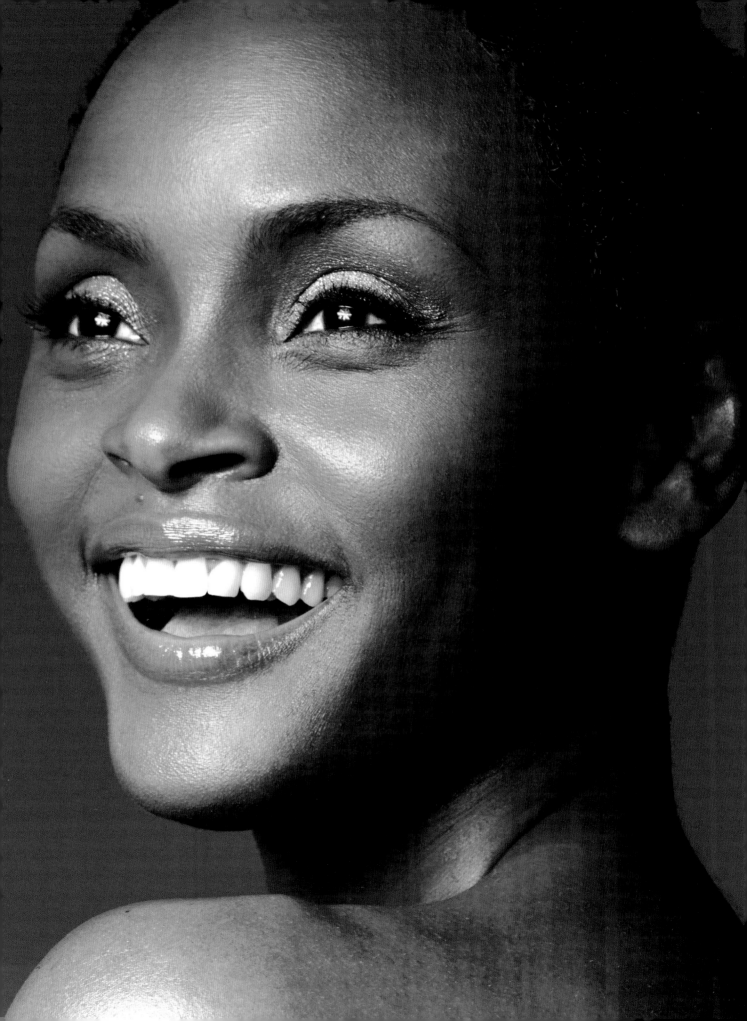

ADDING COLOR TO THE CHEEKS FOR A YOUTHFUL LOOK

Blush can make all the difference in creating a healthy, youthful-looking face. As a general guideline, for a natural look keep cheek color to a minimum so that the focus will be on other areas like the lips or eyes.

CHOOSING A COLOR

If you have a darker skin tone, your blush shade should be slightly brighter; if you have a lighter skin tone, it should be soft and sheer. Blushes with a slightly pink undertone work best, as they duplicate the flushed look the skin gets after a workout. You can also incorporate more warm colors like peaches to create different makeup looks.

Pale
Keep colors light and matte for the most natural look. Try soft peach or pale rose.

Medium
Look to warm pinks or peachy pinks that work with almost any makeup such as pinky-peach, salmon, and candy pink.

Olive
As skin gets darker, look for darker and brighter colors, but apply with a soft touch to get just a hint of color. Look for peachy-pink with shimmer or candy pink with shimmer.

Honey
Bright peaches and dark pinks with shimmer look lovely against warm skin.

Caramel
Coral, apricot, and persimmon shades will show up beautifully against dark skin.

Ebony
Choose brighter and more intense and pure colors like raspberry or oranges.

ROSACEA

Blush may not be necessary; however, cancelling out uneven cheek coloring with foundation or concealer, then applying a uniform blush in a pale tone can give the skin a balanced, natural look without adding redness. Choose matte blushes with minimal shimmer and neutral colors.

TO CREATE A FULLER FACE

Keep contouring shades to the outer borders of the face and apply blush to the apples of the cheeks, blending slightly farther out to cover a larger surface area. Avoid dropping color below the cheekbone.

Nude eyes + bright cheeks + nude or neutral lips
= fresh look

ADDING HIGHLIGHTER

Use cream or powder highlighter to add dimension to the cheeks. Luminosity at the lower temples and slightly above the outer cheeks gives the illusion of lifted cheekbones.

Apply blush to the apples of the cheeks to add youthfulness and a healthy glow to the face. For very sallow skin, you can also apply to the temples and chin. To thin out the face, use contour not blush. Blush should be used to add color; contour should be used to create dimension.

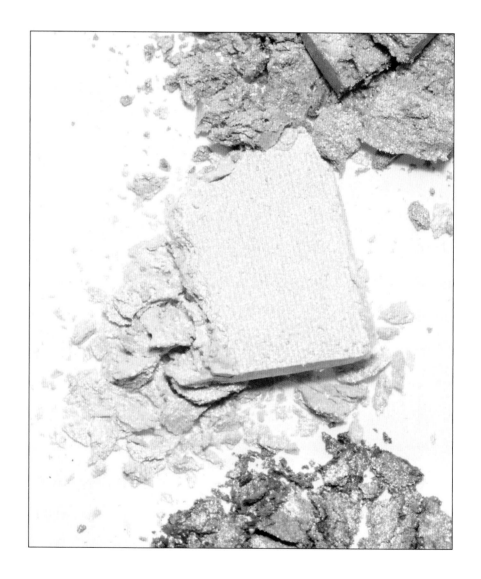

THE ULTIMATE BLUSH

Contour + bronzer + blush + highlight =
the ultimate formula to create dimension, while still
keeping your face soft and pretty

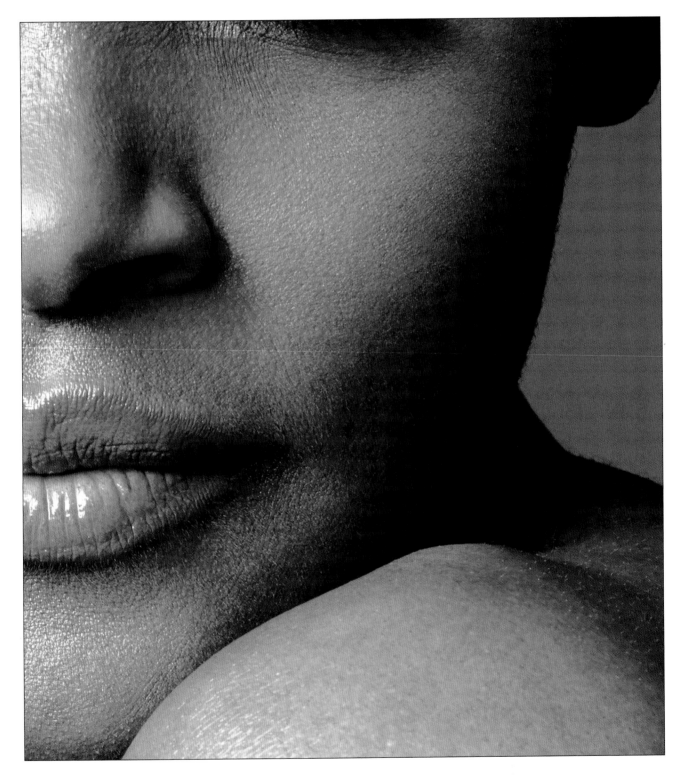

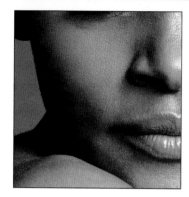

Blush for Darker Skin

1. Apply a chestnut stick foundation to the face and neck.
2. Contour using an espresso stick foundation to the outside edges of the face, the temples, the cheeks, sides of the nose, and under the jawline.
3. Apply a cream concealer in chestnut.
4. Set foundation using a terra-cotta-colored loose powder.
5. Apply a bright persimmon-colored powder blush at the apples of the cheeks.

EYES

1. Apply light shimmering gold eye shadow to the base of the lid and along the bottom lash line.
2. Apply deep brown eye shadow to the outside corners of the eyes and bottom lash line.
3. Apply black cream eyeliner along the top of the lash line and at a 45-degree angle at the outside corners of the eyes.

LASHES

1. Apply two coats of volumizing mascara to the top and bottom lash lines.
2. Apply half or corner black false eyelashes to the outside corners of the eyes.

BROWS

1. Apply dark brown eyebrow powder along the tops of brows and lightly fill in the sparse areas and to the tails.

LIPS

1. Apply chestnut lip liner along the entire natural lip line and fill in with a few dashes.
2. Apply rosy-beige lipstick to the entire mouth covering the lip liner.
3. Apply a shimmering sheer peach lip gloss to the center of the mouth.

Blush for Lighter Skin

Natural and matte

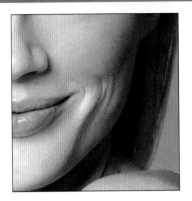

SKIN

1. Apply a beige foundation all over the face and neck.
2. Contour lightly using a warm brown foundation on the outside edges of the face, the temples, the cheeks, sides of the nose, and under the jawline.
3. Set foundation using a translucent loose powder.
4. Apply light brown bronzer along the cheekbones and temples.
5. Apply matte pale peach blush at the apples of the cheeks.

EYES

1. Apply pale shimmering gold eye shadow to the base of the lid.
2. Apply dark brown eye shadow to the outside corners of the eyes.
3. Apply black cream eyeliner along the top of the lash lines and at a 45-degree angle at the outside corners of the eyes.

LASHES

1. Curl eyelashes at the base, middle, and tips.
2. Apply two coats of black mascara to the top and bottom lash lines.
3. Apply individual false eyelashes to the entire top lash lines.

BROWS

1. Apply light-ash-brown brow powder along the tops of brows and lightly fill in the sparse areas. Apply a medium-ash-brown to brow tails.

LIPS

1. Apply nude lip liner slightly above the natural lip line.
2. Apply a pinky-beige lipstick to the entire mouth, covering the lip liner.
3. Apply clear lip gloss to the center of the mouth.

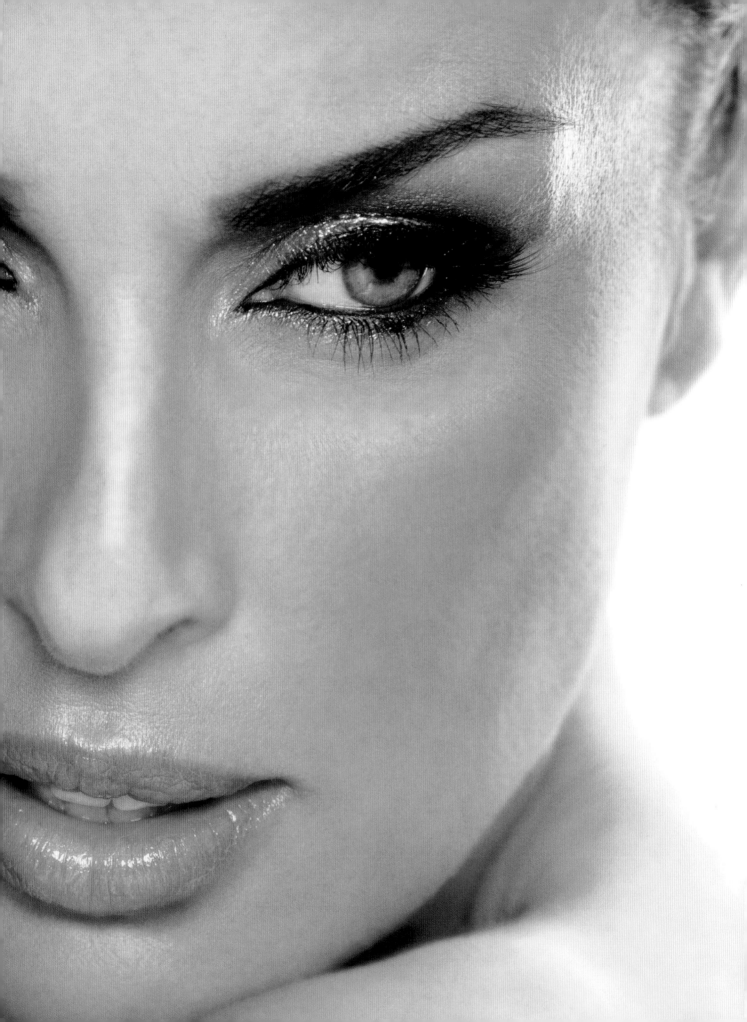

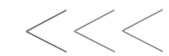

EYES

Common Challenges and How to Fix Them

Eyes are such an important focal point and yet the first to show signs of aging, as they are covered by the thinnest layer of skin on the face. They tell you so much about a person: if she had a bad night's sleep, what kind of mood she's in, even what side of her face she regularly sleeps on. I prefer eyes to tell a different story, one of empowerment. Throughout my travels, however, I have discovered that for most women, eyes are the most difficult part of their makeup routine. "How do I do my eye makeup?" is the number one question I'm asked. When I asked, "Well, what are you looking to do?" the answer more often than not is, "I just want them to look like how they did before." I completely understand. They mean before the brows and eyelids began to droop and when the eyeliner used to glide on smoothly. When your eyes are well done, you can appear more alert, vibrant, and feel confident when someone looks at you. You're able to use your eyes to communicate more effectively, and it completes the overall look of how you want the world to see you.

EYE SOLUTIONS

HOODED LIDS

The skin around the eyes is significantly thinner than the rest of the skin on our face. As we age, collagen breaks down in the already thin skin and causes it to sag, creating a hooded effect or the lid folding onto the lash line. Start combating these effects early with eye creams and sunscreens. Even wearing foundation on the eyelids will provide some level of protection. Hooded lids can cause liners and mascaras to smudge. To battle raccoon eyes, use waterproof eyeliners and mascaras to minimize this effect. Use waterproof eye makeup remover to thoroughly clean eyes at the end of the day.

PUFFY EYES

The appearance of puffiness can be due to the swelling of tissues around the eyes caused by fluid retention. It can also be caused, however, by loose skin and falling fat. The collagen breakdown of the layer of tissue that holds the fat in the eye area weakens and causes drooping and sagging. To minimize the risk of this, use antiaging eye creams and sunscreens. Avoid rubbing the delicate eye area, and sleep on your back, elevating your head slightly whenever possible to prevent fluid from accumulating while you sleep .

FINE LINES

As we get older, cell turnover slows and dead skin cells build up around the eyes. The skin thins and collagen breaks down, reducing the elasticity in the skin and causing lines. Fine lines can be minimized by using eye creams and eye masks that promote cell turnover and help rebuild collagen. Our cells regenerate while we sleep so make sure to apply eye creams in the evenings and sunscreens specified for eye areas in the mornings.

VEINS

Visible veins in the eyes can be the result of irritation from cosmetics, environmental factors like smog or allergens, or lack of sleep. To reduce the appearance of veined or bloodshot eyes make sure all old makeup is removed and use eye drops to clear and flush out eyes. If this happens during the day when makeup is already applied, use drops and hold a tissue along the bottom lash line to allow any debris to flush out without ruining makeup. In any case, the health of your eyes is most important. If you need to remove all eye makeup and start again, it may be the best option for irritated eyes.

Apply foundation or concealer on eyelids to hide any visible capillaries and avoid pink or purple eye shadows.

MILIA

Milia are dead skin cells that get caught in pores and trapped by a layer of skin, creating white bumps that are often found on lids and under eyes. They are caused by several factors: heredity, sun exposure, and heavy creams. To minimize and prevent milia, exfoliate the skin under the eyes using eye creams and masks that contain gentle exfoliating acids, retinols, and/or vitamin C. Use sunscreen, eye creams, or serums that are lighter in texture and avoid thicker creams not specifically formulated for the eye area.

SUN DAMAGE

The sun is a big contributor to most eye area problems. Darkness, fine lines, and milia all worsen with sun exposure. To minimize effects of the sun, make sure to always use sunscreen. One designed for the eye area is best. During summer months or on especially bright days wear sunglasses that have both UVA and UVB protection for added protection of both the skin around the eyes as well as the retina. During prolonged periods of sun exposure, like long walks, gardening, or days on the beach, add hats to your ensemble to protect eyes and skin. Makeup will also add a physical barrier so make sure to add foundation or concealer as well as shadow to eyelids for added protection.

OILY EYELIDS

Women with oily lids tend not to get as many fine lines or wrinkles but can still have significant sagging with age if they don't protect and take care of thinning eyelids. It can also be difficult to wear eye makeup, as the oiliness causes cosmetics to smudge or crease. Waterproof mascaras and eyeliners will minimize any smudging. Dust a layer of silica-based powder on the lids before applying eye shadow to absorb excess oil. Stick concealers tend to take longer to melt so apply a small amount of concealer instead of foundation to lids before makeup. Eye makeup primer is also very useful in keeping shadows and liners from smudging.

SENSITIVE EYES

Eyes can become increasingly more sensitive as we get older. Those with sensitive eyes may be surprised to discover that issues can be solved with proper makeup hygiene and a few simple tips:

- Use saline droppers to keep eyes hydrated.
- Throw out mascara after two to three months.
- If necessary, use disposable mascara wands to avoid contaminating the tube.
- Use plastic makeup scrapers or the back of a clean brush to pick up any products that are in a pot such as cream gels or eye shadows.

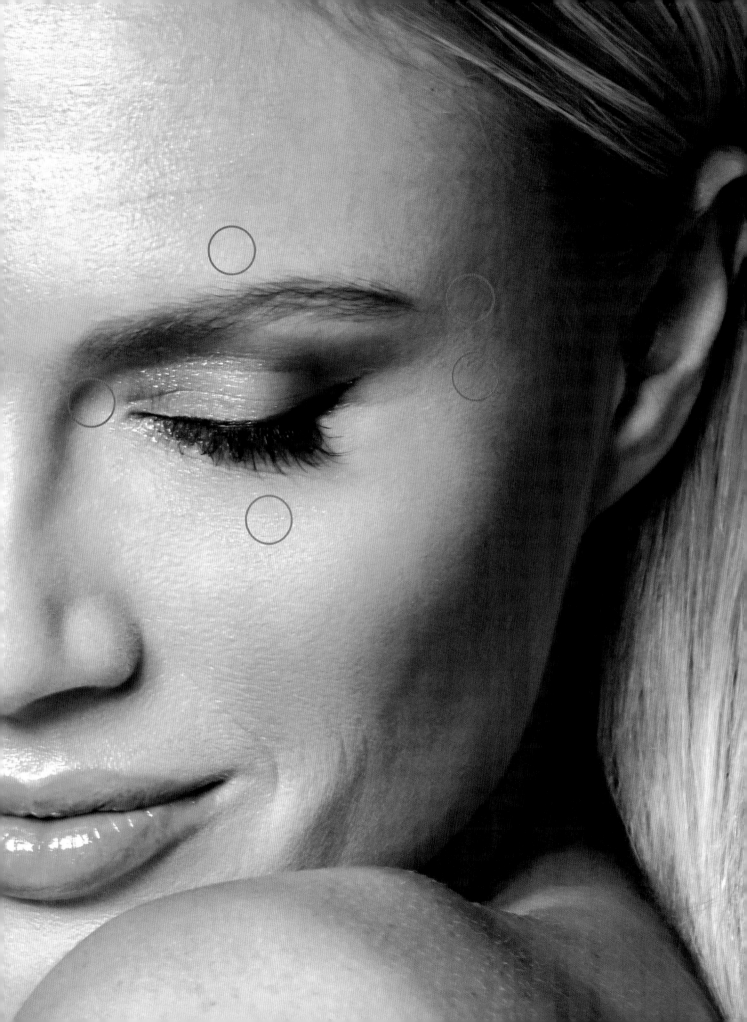

- Sharpen eye pencils before each use to remove any remnants of possible contamination.
- When using twist eyeliners, roll eyeliner on clean tissue paper several times to remove outer layer before and after each use.
- Talk to your ophthalmologist to see if you have a specific allergy.
- Don't apply moisturizers too close to the eye. The skin will absorb eye creams and moisturizers into a larger surface area than originally applied so it may bleed into the eyes if the moisturizer is applied too close.
- Avoid glitter and flakey mascaras, which can fall into eyes and irritate them further.
- Avoid hard and waxy eyeliners. Splurge on softer products for around the eye area.
- If you tend to get a lot of shadow in your eye, try a cream-to-powder eye shadow or use an eye makeup primer before application.
- Look for hypoallergenic makeup, which is ophthalmologist-tested for sensitive eyes.
- If your eyes tend to tear, use waterproof gel eyeliners and mascaras.
- Remove makeup thoroughly with waterproof eye makeup remover.
- If you tend to blink uncontrollably during makeup application, hold the lid you are working on down by gently stretching the skin at the outside corner of your eye out toward your temples using your opposite hand.

DARKNESS

Dark circles, which tend to become more pronounced as we age, are often caused by thin skin. This results in visible blood vessels or excessive melanin (skin pigment) production in the affected area. But whether your under-eye "bags" are hereditary or a result of your lifestyle or environment, these simple tips can help reduce them:

- Eye masks that contain vitamin C as well as vitamin K are a great way to minimize dark circles. They inhibit melanin production for those who have dark circles due to natural pigmentation.
- Sunscreen-infused eye creams are crucial to protect the under-eye area from sun exposure. The sun thins out already thin skin under the eyes; sunscreen helps to minimize further thinning of the skin, as well as future darkness that can be caused by tanning under the eyes.
- Brighteners are great for instant gratification. They have reflective properties that lighten up the eye, and often contain mica to add a slight shimmer to the under-eye area. Wear underneath concealer.
- Sleeping (preferably on your back) is probably the most effective method of reducing dark circles. Keeping the head slightly elevated reduces swelling of tissues and veins. Sleeping on your side can also push on thin skin around the eye area, creating unnecessary damage. Cells heal at night so give your eyes a break and get your eight hours.
- Cold cucumbers placed over the eyes are a natural astringent and shrink and constrict the body tissues.

- Black tea contains tannic acid and caffeine, which constrict vessels to minimize any dark under-eye veins. Tea bags may stain light or very dry skin, however, so moisturize before applying cold tea bags to eyes.
- Exercise will increase circulation and pump oxygen into the vessels, which will increase blood flow. This is important as often dark circles are caused by veins not getting enough oxygen.
- Vitamins, particularly iron supplements, can be effective. Iron deficiencies will often cause dark circles. Try iron in a liquid rather than pill form to help control iron loss and get more oxygen into the veins.
- Water will flush out toxins in your body that can cause dark circles, so be sure to drink plenty of it.

CIRCULATION

Avoid splashing your eyes with very cold or very hot water or rubbing your eyes when you're tired—either of these actions can increase fine lines and break capillaries. Try a pressure-point massage instead. This has been a part of Eastern medicine for centuries and is a great way to improve circulation in the eye area. Using your middle fingers, gently apply pressure to the pressure-point areas around your orbital bone and hold each pressure point—middle of the brow bone, the upper and lower temple, middle of the top of the cheek bone, and along the sides of the nose near the inner corner of your eyes—for three to five seconds. Begin above the brows and repeat as necessary. Try this for instant relief instead of rubbing your eyes or if you have a headache. Remember, too, to take long, slow breaths to simultaneously minimize stress.

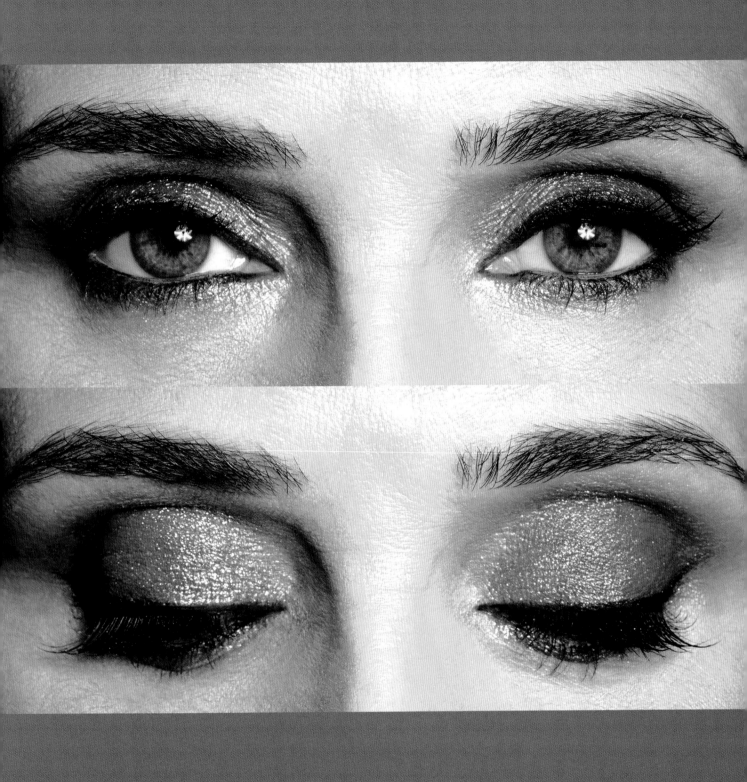

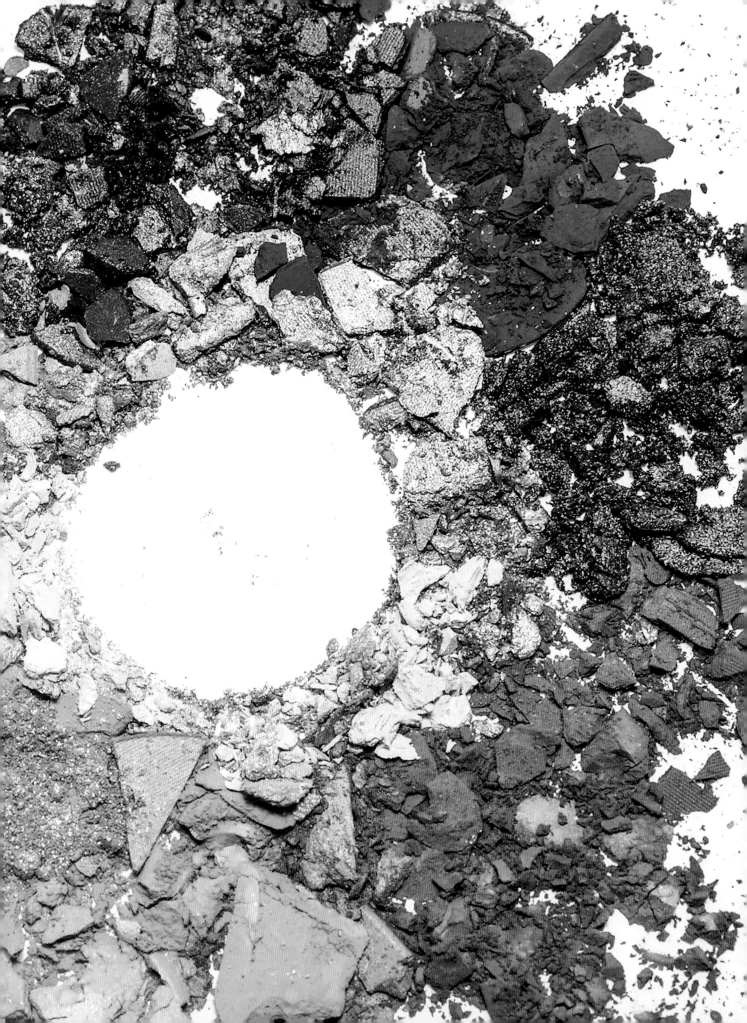

EYE SHADOWS

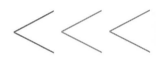

Your eyes are ever changing, especially after age forty. The collagen and elastin break down, causing lids to sag and change textures. Lashes may fall out due to hormone changes, and brows will become increasingly sparser. You may need different liners for changing textures on the eyelids and brighter shadows. While shades of brown can be the most natural-looking and safe choice, browns can make sallowing skin appear to be flat and lifeless. Add shimmers to your brown routine or consider adding new colors like mauve, navy, warm olive, opal, or gold to add vibrancy to the eyes.

To make eye shadows last longer, prime lids with a little foundation and a light dusting of powder. This ensures a smooth application of eye shadow as well as an evening out of any discoloration on the eyelids, allowing the eyes to appear vibrant and closer to their true hue.

There are several differences between a low-quality eye shadow versus a high-quality eye shadow. This is important especially when it comes to aging lids. First consider the actual texture: Is it chalky, which can sit in fine lines, or is it silky smooth? Is the color uniform throughout, suggesting that it's finely milled, or does it apply heavier on certain areas? Is it lightly shimmery, which can add life to aging eyes or does it have chunks of glitter, which can make eyes appear dated? Good-quality eye shadows are silky and glide on smoothly and can also have the slightest pearliness to them.

Technology today has greatly improved eye shadows since our first introduction to them. In the past eye shadows and chalk shared many of the same ingredients. Today eye shadows contain antioxidants to protect our eyelids from environmental damage, better blending properties, finer shimmers, and an endless choice of colors and application types.

TYPES OF EYE SHADOW

CREAM SHADOW

Creams come in sheer to opaque and are easy to apply. They are best applied with your fingers as your body heat helps to soften the shadow for a smoother application, or for better control, use a sable brush or synthetic concealer or eye shadow brush. Creams are great for natural looks and work best alone or with cream eyeliners. Choose creams with key words like *stay put* or *creaseless*, preferably that are heavily pigmented, which allows you to use minimal product. Cream shadows can give the lids a glowing effect and may be a great alternative for those with very dry lids.

PRESSED SHADOW

When using multiple shades on the lid, pressed shadows are best for layering, not to mention they come in every different color and texture from sheer shimmers to opaque matte black. You can even find them with green tea extracts and antioxidants. Look for finely milled shadows that are silky and soft in texture. Shimmers will work best on the base of the lids as well as inner corner to brighten irises. Use darker contour shadow in matte finishes to create depth and redefine the shape of aging eyes.

STICK/CRAYON SHADOW

These are basically cream shadows in stick form but some do have a tendency to be a little denser in texture because of the form they have to hold. I'm a big fan when I have only two minutes to put on my eye makeup. They're great for speedy, on-the-go application of shadows. They can be used on oily or dry lids. I've found that the ones in pots do tend to stay on longer. Use your finger to blend or a sable or taklon brush if necessary.

CREAM TO POWDER

Longer lasting than cream shadow, cream to powder starts as an easy-to-blend cream and sets to a powder. It's great for those who have dry to oily lids but want a cream shadow for speedy application and a sheer shadow look. It gives the eyes the illusion of a wash of color.

MINERAL SHADOW

Although often limited in colors and textures, shadows that are made with loose minerals can work on oily lids as well as dry lids, but can often appear flat because of their mineral content. Add shimmer to the inner corners of the eyes to add highlight. On the plus side, many of them do have higher SPF compared to other eye shadows, which is essential to help protect eyelids from aging UV rays.

SHADOW FOR AGING EYES

LAYERING

Not all eyes should have the contour shade applied at the outer corners or above the crease to create depth, such as those who have no crease (monolids) or very thin lids. Use the following layering technique for these issues as well as small eyes, hooded lids, a short distance between the lashes and eyebrows (often those with very full eyebrows) or if you need a simplified makeup look. To create depth and shape in eyes, work in layers similar to a rainbow, applying the lightest color first at the base of the lid below the brow bone and begin layering contour colors with the darkest color closest to the lash line. You can apply one color of shadow or multiple layers.

Use eyeliner as it helps define the lash line as well as the shape of your eyes, a key item for aging eyes to give the illusion of lift to falling lids or to create bigger eyes.

Base Color

The base color is the primary shade of your eye makeup look. The undertones of the highlight and contour color will complement this shade. Apply it to the base of the lid and along the bottom lash line (optional), omitting the brow bone area.

Highlight (A Shade Lighter Than Your Skin Tone)

Add highlight to your shadow look to brighten the eye area. It adds luminosity to dark, smokey eyes, which otherwise can look harsh and brings deep-set features forward. Choose colors with the same undertones as the base color. Try opal for cool colors or soft gold for warm colors. Avoid intense shimmer for a more natural look. Apply to the inner corners, along the bottom lash line, or try under the base color to add dimension to flat lids.

The more layers you use the more dramatic the look. Make sure to always slightly blend the layers together carefully as to not completely mix the colors together. Mixing colors may cause the shadows to appear muddy.

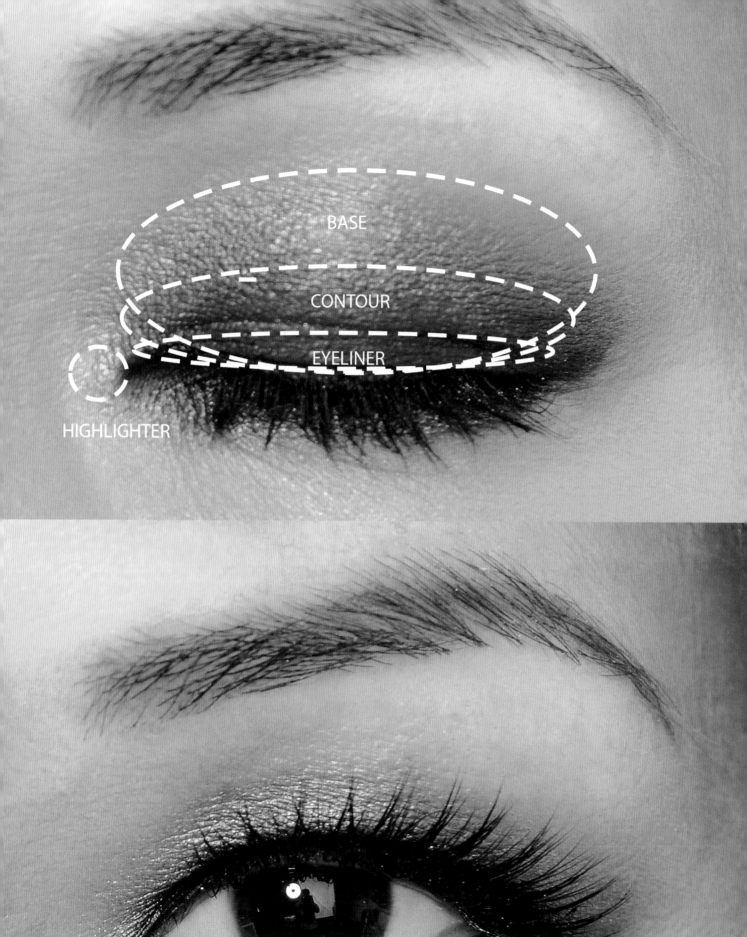

BASE

CONTOUR

EYELINER

HIGHLIGHTER

Contour Color (A Shade Darker Than Your Skin Tone)

The contour shade adds depth to the eyes. When layering shadows, apply contour color on top of other shadow colors but close to the base of the eyes near the lash line to create depth. Make sure to apply it thick enough to be visible when the eyes are open. For hooded lids it may be necessary to apply a slightly thicker layer to the outside corners of the eyes to be visible. This does not mean to create a > shape on the corner as with contouring, more similar to a filled triangle.

Eyeliner

The final step in the layering application, eyeliner adds definition and shape to the eyes. (See eyeliner tips, page 75.) Apply after eye shadows for intense color, or soften the line by using dark shadow as your liner.

Before starting any great eye-makeup application, be sure to examine and prep the skin. This ensures that you'll get the smoothest application possible and minimize imperfections in the skin like fine lines or spots.

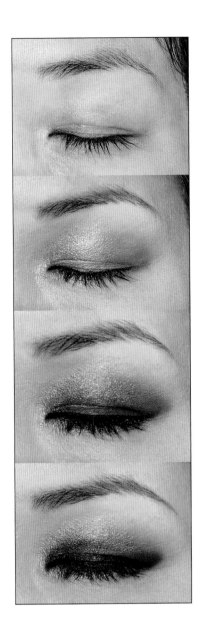

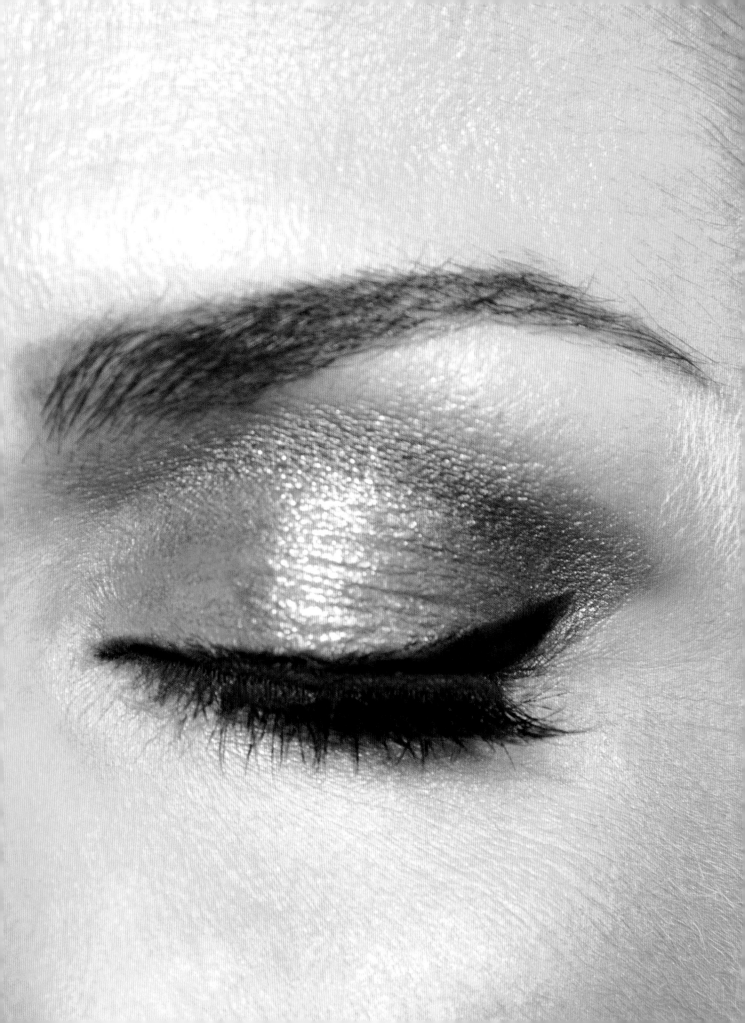

CONTOURING

Contouring is opening up the eye by applying a dark contouring shade above your natural crease and a highlight shade at the center of the lid to create the illusion of larger eyelid space. To give the appearance of wider eyes, you can extend the outer corners of the eyes using a contour shade farther out past the natural end of the eyes.

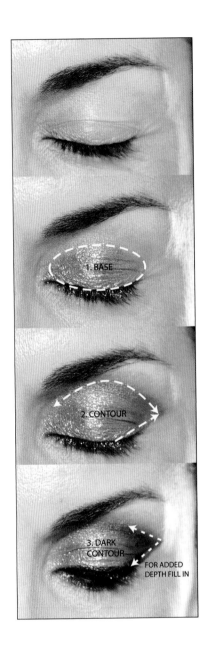

BASE COLOR

The base color is the primary shade of your eye-makeup look. The undertones of the highlight and contour color will complement this shade. Apply it to the base of the lid and along the bottom lash line (optional), omitting the brow bone area.

HIGHLIGHT (A SHADE LIGHTER THAN YOUR SKIN TONE)

Add highlight to your shadow look to brighten the eye area and create the appearance of a larger lid space. Highlighting shadows add luminosity to dark, smokey eyes, which otherwise can look harsh, and brings forward features that are deep set. Choose colors with the same undertones as the base color. Try opal for cool colors or soft gold for warm colors. Avoid intense shimmer or glitter for a more natural look. Apply to the inner corners along the bottom lash line or try in the center of the base of the eyelid to add dimension and open up the eyes.

CONTOUR COLOR (A SHADE DARKER THAN YOUR SKIN TONE)

The contour shade adds depth to the eyes. Apply contour on top of other shadow colors but above the crease, and connect the outside corners. Apply the contour shade at a 45-degree angle to redefine shadows and to lift and lengthen lids. Look for contour colors with a matte finish to create more depth. Avoid mixing shimmery highlight and glittery contour colors.

EYELINER

The final step in contouring makeup application, eyeliner adds definition and shape to the eyes. (See eyeliner tips, page 75.) Apply after shadows.

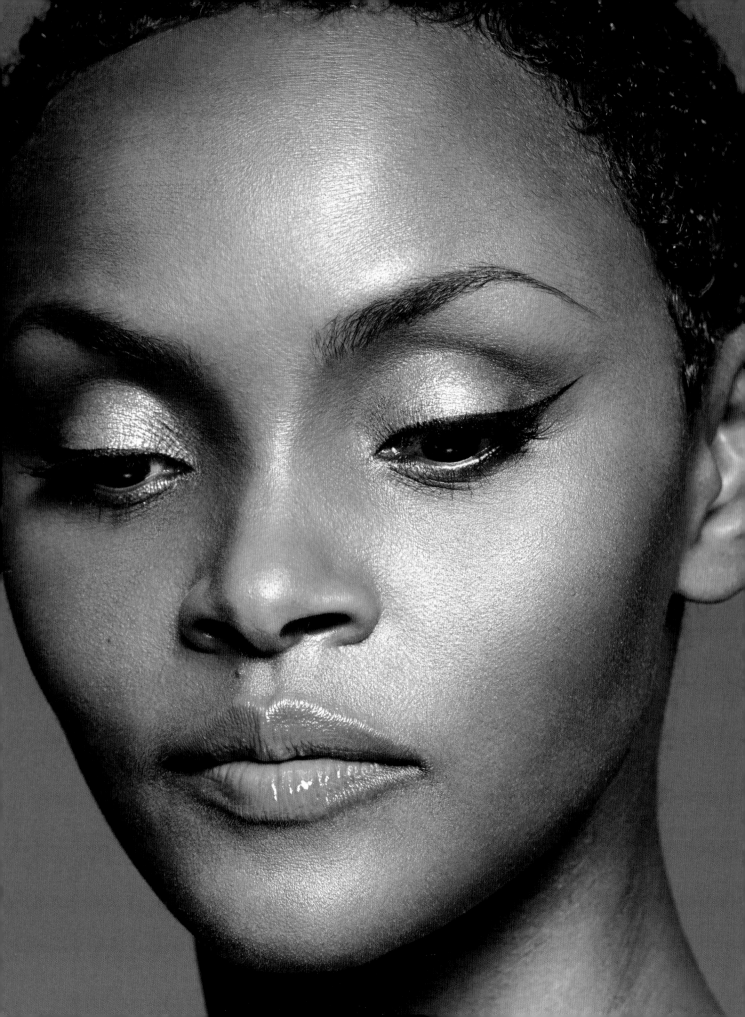

INSTANT EYELIFT WITH EYELINER

One of the most essential techniques to learn is eyeliner application for aging eyes. Simply following the line of your top lids can actually exaggerate the "fall" if you don't angle the end of the line upward. Applying eyeliner at the right angle can make the most dramatic difference in the shape and look of eyes. It is important when applying eyeliner that you consider your eye shape in relation to your face. Are your eyes close set? If so, begin the eyeliner application no closer than where the iris begins and extend liner out slightly past the outside corners to give the illusion of wider-set eyes. Applying too much liner along the lower lash line can drag eyes down; instead, make sure to focus on the top lash line to give the illusion of "taller" eyes. Think of liner as a magic pen and apply where you want fullness and at an angle where you want to see lift.

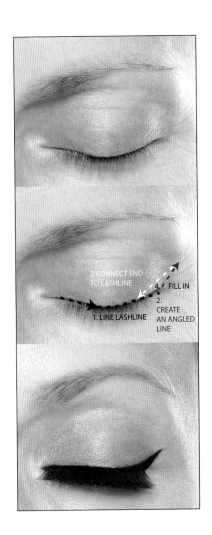

EYELINER TIPS

- Apply dark brown, dark gray, or black eyeliner on the upper outer corners of the eyes at a 45-degree angle to create the illusion of lift.
- Try gel cream eyeliners in a pot.
- Look for smudge-proof or waterproof liners; they often come in twist form.
- For cream liners or gel liners, use a soft, small, detailed eye shadow brush in sable or taklon for the best results.

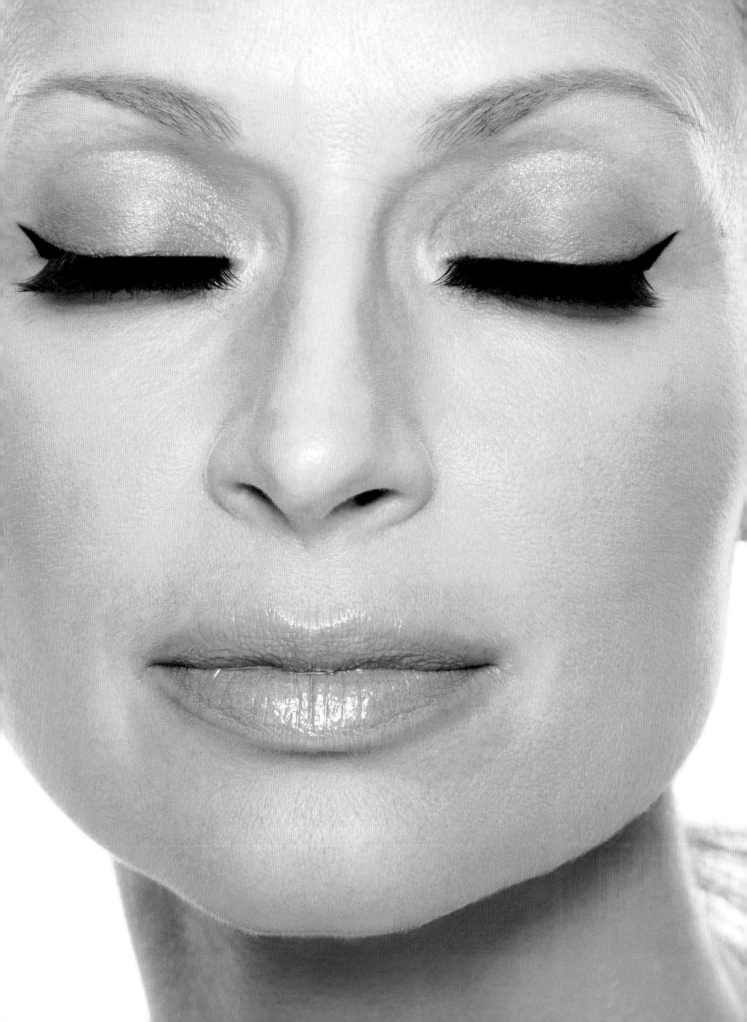

APPLICATION METHODS

These eyeliner application techniques will "bring the eye up." Whether you are creating a natural look or a smokey eye, they will minimize droopiness in the lids (specifically the outer corners), making the eyes appear more youthful and awake.

HOW TO LIFT OUTER CORNERS

Apply eyeliner at the outside corners of the eyes beginning at a 45-degree angle and slightly extending the line to make eyes look wider and lifted. For eyes that are sagging, the angle may need to be even more vertical. The line at the outside corners can be as thick as you need for it to be seen.

TOP-LID APPLICATION

Apply eyeliner along the top lash line for a natural look that is still defined. Apply a thin line of black eyeliner on the top lid as close to the lash line as possible. For close-set eyes, it's important to slightly extend the liner to draw the eyes farther out and begin the line slightly outside the inner corner.

Smokey

Here, eyeliner is applied on the top and bottom lids and blended out. If the lines are smudged slightly, applying eyeliner around the entire eye will give the illusion of larger eyes. Make sure to lift outside corners, and opt for dark browns or slate for a softer look.

LOWER EYELINER

Applying a small amount of liner to the lower lash lines can add definition and sultriness to eyes. Applying too much can make eyes appear to be sagging. As a general rule, make sure the line on the lower lash line is thinner than the line on the top lash line, to create a defined, but still youthful, look.

Thick

Applying a thick amount of liner to the top lid will give lots of lift to eyes but also a slight vintage look. The eye will be drawn to wherever eyeliner is applied. This look is also great for thin or monolids who need to add more height to the eyes as eyeliner helps create whatever shape you want to achieve. Angle at the outer corners to create an even more lifted look.

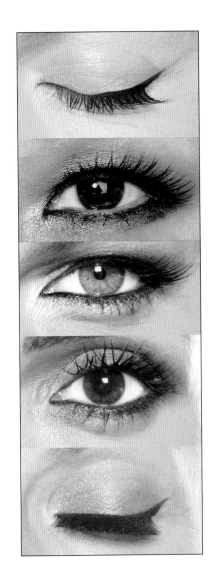

PRODUCTS AND TOOLS

I remember the days when there was only one type of eyeliner in the market; the texture was so hard I thought it was a brow pencil relabeled as eyeliner. It hurt to apply and the pigment was terrible. Technology has changed liners dramatically. Today's liners go on smoothly (essential, to avoid pulling the delicate skin around eyes) and have staying power.

PENCIL EYELINER

Pencil liners should be soft and go on smoothly without any tugging. Avoid pencils that are poorly made, waxy, and hard, as they pull at the skin (which encourages fine lines and wrinkles) and don't deposit enough color. Smudge the line with an eyeliner brush to create sultry, smokey eyes. Set this liner with the same color eye shadow to minimize bleeding, or use waterproof formulas for defined lines that don't smudge or smear.

WATERPROOF EYELINER

Most types of eyeliners are available in waterproof form, which is great for women whose eyes tend to water and cause their makeup to smear. The shape of many aging eyelids are prone to smudging as they can hood over and changing hormones can cause eyes to water periodically throughout the day, particularly along the lower lash line or crease. In addition waterproof eyeliners last longer than other pencils, which means that once you apply it, it will stay on without the need for touch-up. Choose one that goes on smoothly and doesn't pull at the skin around the delicate eye area (usually in a twist pencil tube). Make sure to keep the cap on at all times, as waterproof formulas can dry out faster than other pencil eyeliners.

CREAM EYELINER

Essentially the contents of pencil eyeliner in a pot, cream eyeliner's dense, highly pigmented texture is ideal for maturing eyes as it lines eyes without the skipping that can occur with pencil eyeliners (aging eyelid texture causes the line to appear dotted as it skips over wrinkles). Cream eyeliners are usually available in black, navy, and dark brown but are becoming more widely available in a variety of colors from metallic to charcoal gray. Try it instead of eye shadow to create a cleaner, smokey eye or try a dark-colored cream liner instead of black liner for a softer look. Since cream liner is heavier and dense it tends to last longer. Cream liners come in nice shimmers as well, which is great to create a dramatic look quickly. Look for long-wear formulas and apply using a small sable or taklon brush. Cream eyeliners are usually denser than gel eyeliners and usually have a matte finish.

GEL EYELINER

Gel eyeliner is a great tool to create a perfect, sharp line and also works well for mature women because it gives the eye a lined look without pulling at the delicate skin. It's thinner than a cream eyeliner and has a slightly shinier look. Apply it as quickly but as carefully as possible, as once it's set it doesn't move.

LIQUID EYELINER

Liquid eyeliner comes with a brush or foam applicator to create the thinnest line possible. This allows you to get closest and into the lash line. While larger brushes may be used to create a line at the tops of lashes, a more fine brush will allow you to get in between lashes and create a more defined line. You can also paint the tops of eyelashes using liquid liner to cover up any fallen eye shadow.

BEIGE EYELINER

Look for a creamy texture; you can get away with an inexpensive one for this purpose. Beige is great for the waterline. To brighten and open up tired, red eyes, look for a light beige or pale salmon. Beige eyeliner can also can be used to mark off tweezing areas for eyebrows.

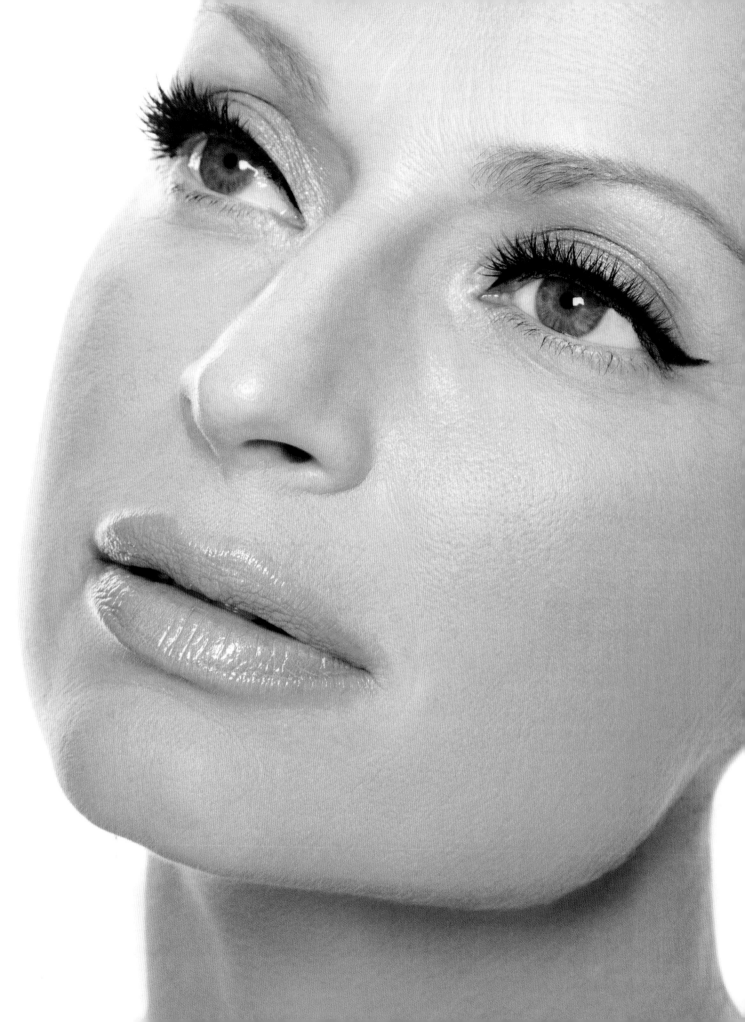

FINISH

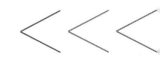

EYELASHES

Lush lashes give eyes the illusion of youthfulness and an irresistible flirty quality, but most important, they can "lift" the eyes open and soften the face.

While we grow a new set of eyelashes every two months in our youth, it is common to lose a significant amount of lashes as we get older. In addition, new lashes come back more sparse than the time before. Use the tips and tricks below to fake youthful fullness.

CHOOSING YOUR MASCARA

When choosing your mascara, first figure out what type of eyelashes you have. Are they sparse, short, or thin? Then find the appropriate mascara that will achieve whatever effect you are looking for—volumizing, lengthening, and so on.

LOOK TO THE WANDS

If the wand bristles are not uniform and go in every direction, they will deposit a lot of mascara for ultimate coverage. If the bristles are separated and long, they will separate the lashes more and create definition. If they are short, they'll reach the finest, shortest hairs; these are good for sparser eyelashes.

STRAIGHT EYELASHES

Straight eyelashes benefit from waterproof mascara to set curled lashes into place. Look for mascara that's dense in color and not dripping from the brush (a sure sign it will weigh down lashes).

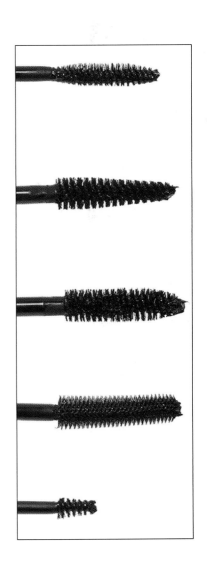

THIN EYELASHES

Look for volumizing mascaras whose wands have bristles of varying lengths that go in random directions, and look for nylon fibers that can adhere to lashes for added thickness.

SHORT EYELASHES

Look for lengthening mascaras whose wands contain nylon fibers to extend lashes.

SHORT, THIN LASHES

Double it up: Apply lengthening mascara then apply volumizing mascara for lashes that need both length and volume. Allow drying time between coats to ensure mascara gets layered correctly and doesn't clump.

ADVANCED LASH-ENHANCING TECHNIQUES

As we age, eyelashes can become sparse or shorten. You can even lose patches of lashes with the onset of menopause. It's important to know what options are available to you should either of these issues arise.

LASH EXTENSIONS

Lash extensions are individual human hairs that are available in varying lengths to the wearer and applied using a strong, permanent adhesive. They are expensive and high-maintenance, but they may be worth the cost for people who don't wear eye makeup daily and have the money and time for upkeep. Hairs can only be adhered onto existing eyelashes so it might not be worthwhile for people with sparse natural lashes. The extensions process must be performed by a professional who has been specially trained to do so. The extensions can be attached to both upper and lower lids. Lash extensions can look so natural that it's difficult to see where the real lashes begin and extensions end. Extensions take a few hours to apply and last about a month; touch-ups also have to be done in between, usually after two weeks for any hairs that may have fallen off or to accommodate for regrowth. Regular touch-ups are necessary if the extensions twist around and can't be pulled off manually. Great care is necessary when working with lash extensions: Makeup that contains any form of oil, including cream shadows, some liners, and mascara cannot be used; be very careful when applying liner and shadow; and never rub your eyes. Sleeping on your back is essential, as lying on either side of your face will cause lashes to twist.

COMMON REASONS FOR EYELASH LOSS

- Alopecia
- Trauma, rubbing eyes
- Pulling out eyelashes (Trichotillomania)
- Mites
- Change in hormones, thyroid, stress

EYELASH TINTING

Vegetable-based dye is applied to lashes to tint them to be more visible, but the dye does not add bulk. Tinting should be done at a reputable salon, as it can cause blindness if performed incorrectly. Women whose lashes have gone gray in sections of their eyes can consider this as an alternative or in addition to mascara as it makes a dramatic difference for 24/7 color. It is also a great alternative to those whose eyes have become increasingly sensitive. Tinting is inexpensive and should be redone every month, as eyelashes naturally fall out and recycle themselves every one to two months.

EYELASH PERMING

Similar to a regular hair perm, lashes are wrapped around tiny perm rods to curl. While lashes stay curly without additional manual curling, there is a significant drawback. Since we get a full set of new lashes every two months, straight lashes appear alongside permed ones in the interim, which creates uneven lashes.

SPECIAL LASH GROWERS

The latest in eyelash technology, these prescription treatments were developed after doctors treating glaucoma patients discovered that one of the side effects of the glaucoma drops were longer, thicker eyelashes. They took the main ingredient, a drug called bimatoprost, and created a cosmetic product that's packaged similar to liquid eyeliner and is applied onto the lash line every evening. These prescription-only products are expensive, with a tube running about $140 for a month supply. The results are significantly better when applied consistently. While non-prescription lash growers (which don't contain bimatoprost) are gaining in popularity, the prescription ones do work better. Whichever type you choose, make sure any lash growers you use are FDA approved.

All lashes are different so it's important to read instructions very carefully, and be aware of side effects—in particular, people with light-colored eyes although rare, may see their eyes become permanently darker. The skin close to the lash line also can be darkened. Also, when product use is stopped lashes can seem sparse.

FALSE EYELASHES

Arguably the biggest secret in beauty is false eyelashes. They are used as widely as lipstick and mascara on the red carpet and on celebrities, but rarely have they trickled down into the mainstream. Even mascara ads are now admitting to the use of false eyelashes in their ads. While the '60s may have deterred modern women from wearing false eyelashes, today's false lashes are almost undetectable from real lashes and can make eyes appear more alert and larger all while retaining a natural look. For aging eyes, false lashes can fill in areas that are sparse or lift outside corners of the eyes that are falling from collagen breakdown. For aging eyes that lack definition, a full strip can lift the eye to make eyes appear open, lifted, and youthful.

How to Keep Eyelashes Healthy

- Eat a quality diet of foods rich in protein and iron to keep hair growth healthy.
- Exercise to keep stress at bay.
- Sleep on your back. Lashes that are lost on one side of the face are more than likely from sleeping on the affected side.
- Clean eyes well with waterproof eye makeup remover. Hold remover onto lids with a cotton ball or pad for several seconds to loosen makeup, and wipe gently to remove all makeup. Never rub eyes. Use a lash conditioner if you have dry, brittle lashes.

FALSE EYELASH STRIPS

Eyelash strips have evolved and can look completely natural, and are very versatile. They come in dozens of different styles. Some offer a retro look while others criss-cross at the base, duplicating the look of natural lashes and are nearly undetectable. It's now hard to tell where natural lashes end and false ones begin. When looking for strips, pay attention to the shape of your eye. Women with wide-set eyes should look for lashes that are longer in the middle of the strip and taper at both ends. This will open up the eyes instead of further widening them. If eyes are more close set, choose lashes that are shorter in the middle and longer at the ends of the lashes. This draws eyes out. When in doubt, try a few different styles to see what works best. Most false eyelash strips need to be cut to fit the length of eyes as all eyes vary in length.

Eyeglass wearers often have a hard time with lashes hitting their lenses, which makes wearing mascara or false eyelashes uncomfortable. Look for shorter false lashes and curl them midway so that the tips bend up. This will prevent them from hitting the lenses.

INDIVIDUAL EYELASHES

Individual lashes create a natural look when falsies are only slightly longer than natural lashes, and are great for women who want very light lash enhancement. Three or four individual lashes on the outside corners to "wing out" the eye or a few in the center to add height and open up the eyes is all that you may need for a natural look. Those with very sparse lashes should stick with strip lashes, as they will hold longer and are easier to apply on a sparse lid. Individual lashes are also great for lash loss to fill in gaps in the lash line.

THREE-QUARTER-STRIP LASHES

These types of strip lashes are shorter than full strips and fit almost every eye. They don't need to be cut.

HALF/CORNER LASHES

These lashes were designed to duplicate the natural look of a combination of a few individual eyelashes without the difficulty of application. They add just a little lift to the ends of eyes and create a natural to dramatic look depending on the length and are a great way to add a little oomph to your lashes without using a complete strip. Ideal for novices and those who may have lost a patch of eyelashes due to hormonal changes or lash trauma and just need some temporary filler.

Applying false eyelashes should be the last step in your routine, as adding any eye makeup on top of false eyelashes can cause them to lift off. For novices, practice applying lashes several times without glue until you're comfortable with the process. The results are well worth the effort.

HOW TO APPLY FALSE EYELASH STRIPS

Once you've found your desired false lashes, you need to cut them to length. To find your perfect eyelash-strip length, without glue, measure strips to the length of your eye, remove, and cut at the outer corners to make the most natural look. Leaving lashes too long will cause them to poke and lift.

Apply glue along the base of the strip. Allow the glue to sit for thirty seconds to get tacky.

Balance the strip on top of eyelashes, attaching false lashes as close to the lash line as possible. (If necessary, use the back of your tweezers or applicator tool to push lashes closer to natural lash line.)

Allow false lashes to dry for fifteen seconds and open eyes gently, making sure that glue has not stuck to the bottom lashes. If it has, use a wet cotton swab and run between top and bottom lashes to remove the glue.

If desired, once glue has dried clear, apply a liquid liner to smooth out the top lash line and cover any remaining glue marks or sheen. Use black or brown liquid eyeliner if necessary to darken the glue line after the glue has dried.

Curl your lashes after you have applied the false lashes. This will allow the false and natural lashes to blend together, making them feel more comfortable.

If you make a mistake, simply remove false lashes, remove the excess glue from the false lashes, and reapply. Remove any glue on your lids if you have any. If some of the glue remains on, don't worry; it will dry clear and be nearly undetectable.

> Cut eyelash strips in thirds to allow for easier application. This allows you to apply them in a connect-the-dot fashion. This is a great solution for those who have a difficult time balancing entire strips on their lashes. Apply on the lash line beginning at the inner corner of the eye and connect from the inner corner to the outer corner. If the last strip is too long, trim accordingly.

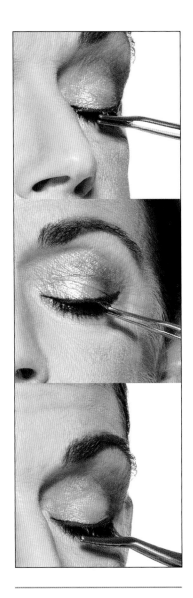

Be careful in choosing the correct lash glue. The glue should not be too runny or too strong—glue that is too strong can make the lashes very painful to remove, which can irritate the delicate eyelid area. Very strong glues tend to be clear and have noticeable fumes when opened.

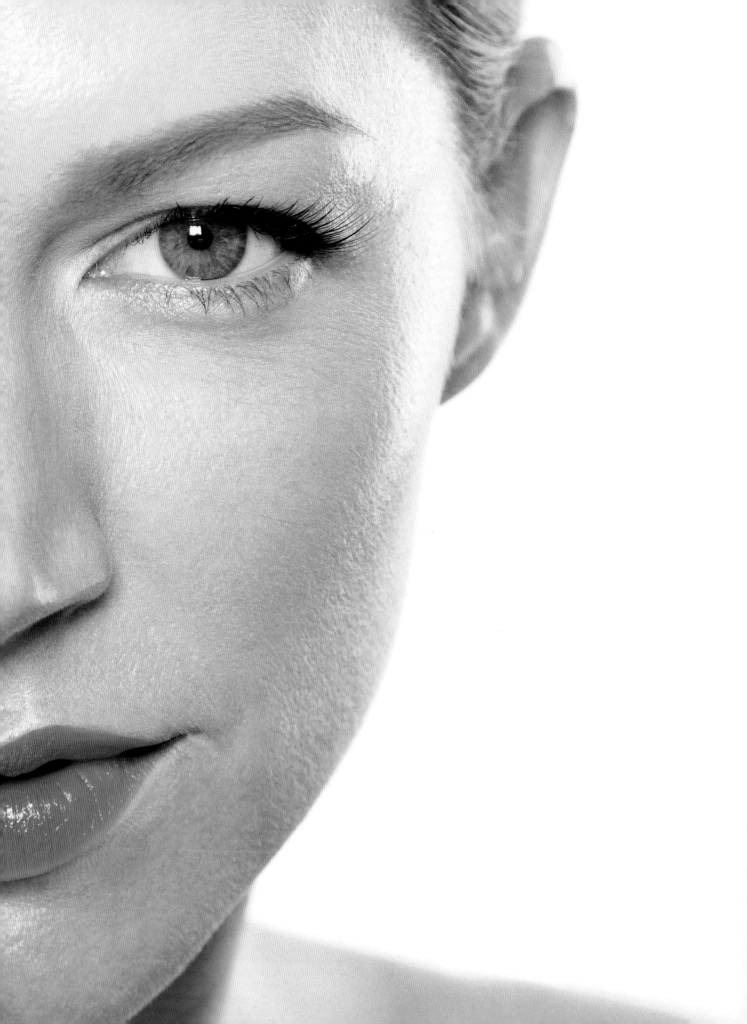

BROW BASICS

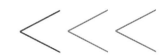

Eyebrows are essential to beautiful eyes. When shaped well, they can add symmetry to not only your eyes but your entire face. They have the capability to make you look softer, polished, and more youthful. Aging eyebrows often have the challenge of falling tails (from a loss of collagen in the forehead) or are often sparse in random areas of the brows. As your eyebrows lose definition, it can be confusing as to how to re-create a new brow or exactly where to tweeze or cut.

Brush brows up to smooth out brow hairs to prepare for cutting and tweezing.

Hairs in aging brows can grow very long and be quite wiry. Cut hairs going against the growth line. Look for scissors with short blades to avoid accidental over-cutting. Use a comb if necessary to hold the hairs in place. If some of the brow hairs grow down and refuse to go up, you can cut them into shape from the bottom as well. Always cut gradually so as to not create holes in the brows.

I prefer to keep the brows as full as possible but beware of stray hairs, which can appear unkempt and unruly. Tweeze above where the brows may start to connect to the hairline. It's important to tweeze underneath the brows, as strays can give the illusion that they're sagging. You can use a white eyeliner to determine tweezing area if you are not sure where to tweeze and need a guide. Cover stray hairs with liner to see how the brows will look once they are tweezed.

BEAUTY TIP

If you wear glasses it can be difficult to tweeze eyebrows. Use a magnifying mirror to tweeze brows as well as a large mirror several times during the process to see how the brows look in relation to your entire face.

CHOOSING YOUR BROW COLOR

Apply a highlighter or eye shadow color or concealer lighter than your natural skin tone right under the brow bone to accentuate the arch in your brows. Choose a matte shade for a natural look or a shimmery color for an evening look.

FILLING IN BROWS

When choosing a brow color to add fullness, consider your natural brow color and add a hint of your hair color to your eyebrows for a uniform look. For example, if you have blond hair and brown eyebrows look for a color that's in between to create flow from your face to hair. A color that is too dark can make you look harsh and create an unwanted frowning effect.

For light hair, you generally want brows to be one to two shades darker than your hair color to create a healthy look.

For dark hair, use one to two shades lighter than your hair color to fill in without creating a harsh look.

For silver hair, use an ashy-brown or gray color to blend with the gray hair.

EXTENDING THE BROWS

With aging, the tails of eyebrows are often the first hairs to go, causing brows to appear shorter and as though they are falling. To create the illusion of an extended brow, choose a color that is slightly darker than your natural brow hairs and never too warm in color and fill in from the top of the arch to redirect the arch to appear higher. Then extend out. You should also fill in any large holes in the brows using this darker color, but not at the beginning of the brows. When using a pencil, use light and gentle strokes for the start of eyebrows and more pressure for the tails of brows to get a similar effect.

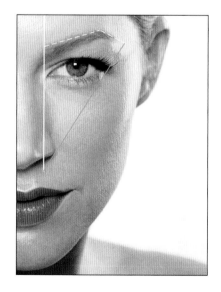

1. Brows should start above the inner corners of the eyes.
   - Hold a pencil on the side of nose and inner corner of the eye. If your brow does not touch the pencil, fill in lightly with a brow pencil or pomade, using short, hairlike strokes.
   - For wide-set eyes, start slightly closer to the bridge of the nose.
   - For close-set eyes, start eyebrows slightly farther out.
2. The arch should start above the outside of the pupil. Aging brows often start to begin falling here. Fill in above the arch to create the illusion of a lifted brow
3. Hold pencil at an angle from the side of the nose to the outside corners of the eyes. The tails of eyebrows should end here. Aging, however, often causes the tails of brows to thin out and become shorter. If brows do not extend to the pencil, use a shade darker than your brow color to extend the ends.

BROW REMOVAL

THREADING

If you are going to opt for a salon brow treatment, threading may be a great option as it does not involve wax, which can exfoliate the already thinning skin around the eye area. A popular method in the East, threading uses simple strings intricately placed to crisscross and remove unwanted hairs. Many people swear it is less painful than tweezing. Make sure to go to a reputable salon, however; I've seen some less-than-hygienic technicians hold the string in their mouths prior to use.

TWEEZING

While tweezing may take more time to complete than other methods of brow removal, it is a great option for aging brows as you can be picky about each and every hair. You want to save as many hairs as you can when you get older and tweeze only what is necessary. Tweezing gives you the luxury of taking time and being precise. Look for high-end tweezers where the tips close completely.

WAXING

The skin around the eye area is so delicate that waxing can be too stripping for the thinnest skin on the face. Sometimes it's the only option, however, as waxing removes hairs quickly and even pulls the smallest hairs that are not visible to most eyes, which leaves a cleaner look. For the safest results, make sure that the wax your salon uses is specifically for the delicate eye area; the wax should be blue or pink and opaque. Honey-colored clear wax is often for the body and should not be used on the face.

PRODUCTS AND TOOLS

BROW POWDER

This is the best product to create softer-looking brows or to fill in sparse areas to create the illusion of fullness. Use powder at the arch of the brow to create softness and a darker shade at the tail for definition. Powder is best applied with an angled brow brush. As an added use, brow powder can also be used to fill in a sparse hairline where your hair parts.

BROW CREAM/POMADES

Cream creates a sharper, more defined brow. It is especially great for filling in sparse areas of the brows because the cream is more opaque and can give the illusion of duplicate brow hairs. For a more natural look, use the cream sparingly at the beginning of the brow for a softer look, as it packs a powerful punch with just a little product. Save the full application for brow tails. It's best to apply brow cream with a thin, angled brow brush made of synthetic material. Brow cream and pomade are ideal choices post illness to redraw lost brow hair.

BROW PENCIL

Brow pencils generally last longer because they contain waxy ingredients that prevent the color from disappearing when you sweat. Pencils are great for creating definition at the ends of brows. Many brow pencils have spiral brushes or dense angle brushes on the opposite side of the pencil. Use them to brush out any hard lines created by the pencil to create a softer look.

BROW GEL

Brow gels are a great option to color gray hairs in between coloring services. They also can lift eyebrows, especially if they grow downward or have become wiry and are difficult to control. Use the gel sparingly and don't touch your brows after the gels sets, as it tends to flake off. Brow gel is available in several shades to match almost any hair color.

EYEBROW STENCILS

Eyebrow stencils are cutouts of different eyebrow shapes, which you can place over your eyebrows as a guide for what needs to be filled in and what may need to be tweezed. Stencils are ideal for those with complete brow loss, as they can help you to create and fill in brow shapes from scratch.

BROW GROWERS

While often designed for the lash line, lash growers have been effective for regrowing brow hairs in many women. Make sure to find products that are FDA approved and follow package directions.

EASY BROW FIXES

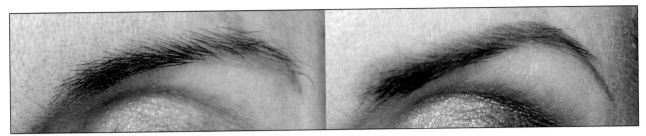

Thin Eyebrows

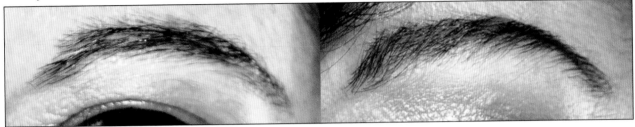

Falling Arches

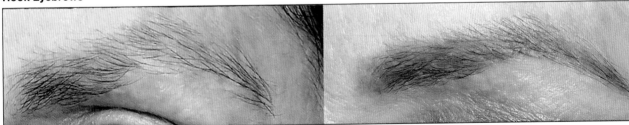

Soft Tails

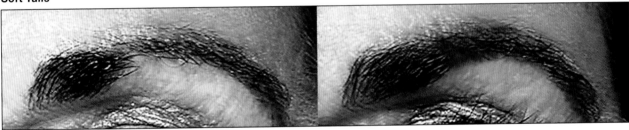

Hook Eyebrows

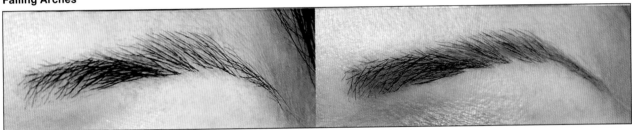

Sparse Eyebrows

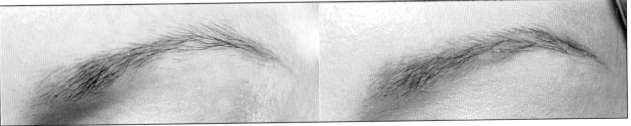

Fine Start

> Work with what you have. For example, if you have thin, rounded eyebrows, fill them in slightly under the arch for a natural look.

THE FURROWED BROW

Too much squinting or worry lines over the years can cause the brows to dip at the inner corners, causing brows to look permanently furrowed. To correct this, keep the area in between the brows clean of any stray hairs. Fill in the tops of brows, starting them slightly farther away from the bridge of the nose.

FALLING ARCHES

The tails of eyebrows are often the first hairs to go as we age, leaving the brow appearing to be falling at the ends with minimal arch. To create the illusion of lift, use your preferred product to draw on top of your natural arch and extend out, creating a tail. It's best to do this in a color slightly darker than your natural brow hairs. I prefer a pomade to deliver more pigment to duplicate the look of dense hairs.

"HOOK" EYEBROWS

Often not knowing where to begin the arch is how the "hook" eyebrow develops. The arch begins too close to the beginning of the brow, and it is a very common error. For aging eyes it creates the look of dark, square corners at the beginning of the eye and a rounded brow, which makes the eyes appear like a hook. Fortunately, the "hook" eyebrow is also one of the easiest to fix. Simply connect the beginning of the brow to the peak of the arch (it should be above the end of the pupil) and fill in. If the eyebrow is too full, tweeze under the beginning of the brow then connect and fill in.

SOFT TAILS

There is a decent amount of shape and fullness throughout the brow but the arches and tails start to lose definition. Use your desired brow filler to lightly fill in the arch and add more pressure to darken the tails.

THIN EYEBROWS

Over-plucking in your youth, when thin eyebrows are the trend, is the cause for this common look. As you age, repeatedly plucked eyebrows rarely grow back, and thin eyebrows can look dated. To stimulate growth, try using brow growers or use an eyebrow pencil powder or pomade and apply color in short, hairlike strokes to duplicate the look of brow hairs. Avoid drawing brows too thick, as this can also look fake.

FINE START

The beginning of the eyebrows are minimal and lack shape, creating the illusion of wider set eyes. Draw a line along the top and bottom of the brows and extend closer to the nose. Fill in only where necessary at the start of the brow using short, soft strokes.

SPARSE EYEBROWS

The entire eyebrow is faint, leaving only a hint of a brow shape. Sparse eyebrows don't frame the face as well as fuller eyebrows, giving an older, sometimes unhealthy effect. To fill in sparse eyebrows draw a line along the top and bottom of the brows and fill in using short strokes to duplicate natural hairs.

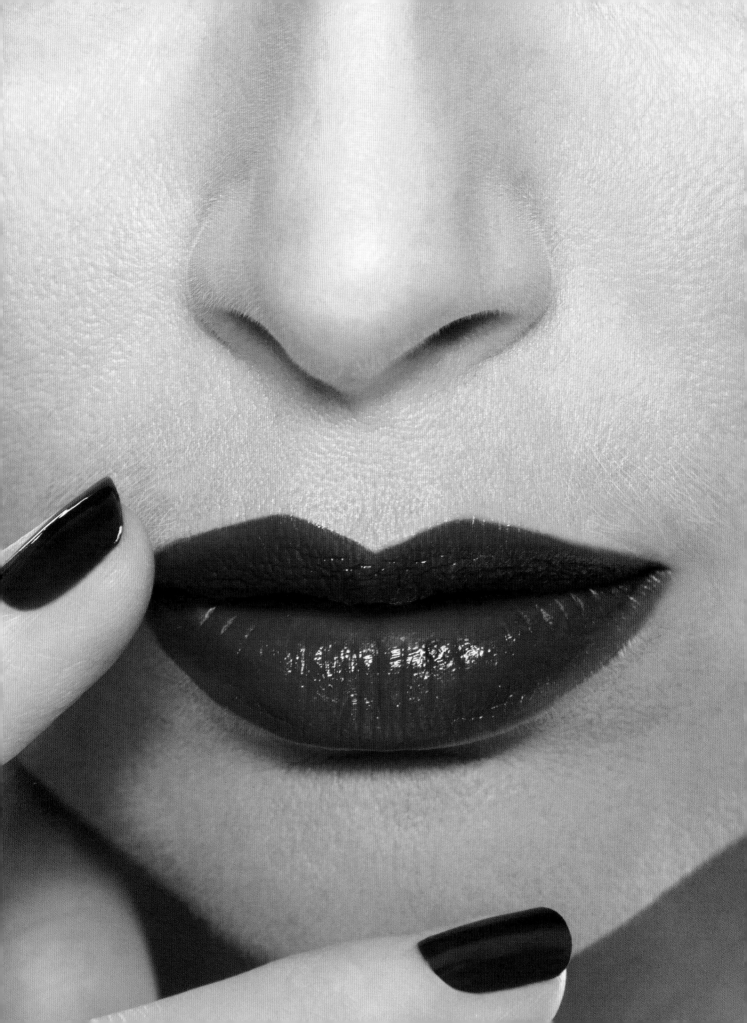

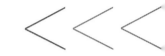

LIPS

Creating the Perfect Pout

Thinning lips are an inevitable issue as we age. Our lips are made of skin only a fraction of the thickness of the skin on our faces. Lips contain no pores or oil glands, which causes them to dry out faster and shrink. Remember, caring for your lips is just as important as caring for your skin!

COMMON ISSUES

SUNBURN

Our lips are just as subject to the damaging rays of the sun as the rest of our face, and sunburn will dehydrate and thin them even more. It is essential to apply balm with broad-spectrum SPF 30-plus on the lips prior to applying any lip color to prevent shrinkage. It's even more important to use lip balm when wearing lip gloss, as gloss typically contains oil-like ingredients and no sunscreen, which can concentrate the sun's rays and burn lips.

CHAPPED LIPS

Apply lip balm to soften loose, chapped skin and use a warm washcloth to gently remove excess skin. Finish with more lip balm. Apply lip conditioner or lip plumper before going to bed, to prevent dryness and keep lips full.

FEATHERING

To minimize feathering, make sure to exfoliate using sugar scrubs specifically designed for the lips or a warm washcloth, Then, moisturize using a lip cream—and don't forget the lip line. This will minimize cracks and grooves. Apply foundation or concealer around the mouth. Lip liner will create the best barrier from feathering. Apply a long-wearing lip color and fill the mouth only in the center with lip gloss if necessary. You can also use a shimmering lip color in a lighter tone at the center of the mouth to create the illusion of depth and gloss.

FAKE IT 'TIL YOU MAKE IT

It's easy to create the illusion of full lips; all it takes is a few tips and tricks to create luscious lips that look like you were born with them.

CREATING A FULLER OUTLINE

Use lip liner to create the illusion of fuller or symmetrical lips. It is important, however, not to go beyond the light highlight that surrounds your lips. Make sure you have no fine hairs close to the lip line, which can appear more defined when darker liner is applied.

When changing the natural lip line to create the illusion of fuller lips, it's important to keep things natural. I prefer a neutral lip liner slightly darker than the natural lip line so that it merely looks like a shadow of your lips. Use lip liners that are one to two shades darker than your natural lip color to redraw the line in a neutral tone.

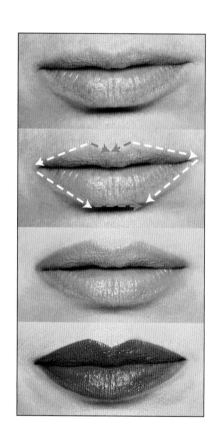

Light skin: nude

Medium skin: light brown

Dark skin: caramel or chestnut

Create fullness to the lips by drawing a V shape, duplicating the Cupid's bow shape (often shrunken on mature lips) on the upper lip line. Then a dash under the center of the bottom lip. Connect the corners, drawing the line slightly above the natural lip line to minimize a larger lower lip to create better balance.

Create width by drawing slightly outside the corners of the mouth to give the illusion of a wider mouth. Slightly fill in the mouth with lip liner.

Apply color.

Apply lipstick on top of liner so that there is no line of demarcation.

Apply gloss just to the center of both the top and bottom lips to give the illusion of full, hydrated lips. This also minimizes bleeding from lip gloss.

Clean up lipstick mistakes or smears with concealer and a small brush to wipe away any smudges.

AROUND THE MOUTH

FACIAL HAIRS

Something we don't ever like to think about is facial hair that emerges as we lose estrogen. But it happens and it's important to check weekly for hairs that have grown along the sides or on and under the chin to keep skin looking smooth and youthful.

MARIONETTE LINES

The lines around our mouth that resemble parenthesis are caused by sagging of the skin as well as the loss of elastin. Highlight the lines using concealer; this will create the illusion of diminished lines. Use masks and moisturizers that contain hyaluronic acid to help plump lines or see a dermatologist about dermal fillers for effects that last from six months to a year. Make sure to follow a proper skin-care regimen to slow the development of marionette lines.

MELASMA (SKIN PIGMENTATION)

Hyperpigmentation or melasma on the upper lip can occur for a number of reasons, many of which are hormonal. Don't be alarmed, as often this is temporary and should greatly subside within time. There are things you can do to conceal the discoloration while it resolves, however, but prevention is key.

Sunscreen is a must on any areas that have darkness since melasma is caused by overactive melanin. Use sunscreen of SPF 30+ and reapply every few hours. Waxing the upper lip with wax not formulated for the face area can cause trauma to the upper lip and remove some skin along with tiny hairs. Pairing this with hormone changes and sun can greatly exaggerate the look and longevity of the darkness. Consider threading as an option if you are finding a lot of darkness on the upper lip and are worried about extra damage to the skin.

Skin bleaching is generally done by applying high percentages (20 percent and above) of hydroquinone to the skin. While this can be very effective at lightening the skin there are very serious side effects. There is a large chance of sensitivity in the area as well as a high chance of long-term uneven pigmentation. Aim for products that contain 2 to 4 percent hydroquinone (the maximum level for over-the-counter products), to ensure gradual, corrective removal of excess pigmentation as opposed to attempting to change your skin's DNA. Always wear sunscreen after.

For aggressive treatments consult a reputable dermatologist before undergoing any procedure.

Cover with Concealer

Apply a full-coverage concealer a half to one shade lighter than your skin tone and with a pink or peach undertone to cancel out melasma's brown undertone. Apply over foundation for an even blend. Avoid using too light a shade of concealer, as this will actually highlight the area.

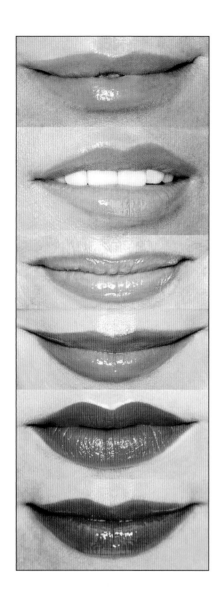

CHOOSING LIP COLORS

- Avoid gold or brown hues, as they can make lips appear drab.
- Frosted lip colors should only be used on the center of the mouth as a highlighter.
- Bold colors like orange, fuchsia, and red should be worn with clean, simple eye makeup and always in matte or satin textures.
- Mauve tones are a great choice for daytime wear on almost any skin tone, with the use of appropriate lip liner.
- Mixing colors is a great way to create new lip colors. Mix warms into cools to deepen or neutralize hues (for instance, beige will warm up pink to create a neutral shade with a hint of color).
- Adding clear lip gloss to boring lip colors can add life to otherwise flat shades.

The darker the eyes, the lighter the lips should be.

- Bold lips are a quick way to make a statement. They should be paired with a clean eye in shimmering highlight colors and liner or light, smokey eyes in gold and bronzes for an evening look.
- Plums in varying shades look great on almost anyone. These can be paired with cool eye shadows in opal, mauve, and purples.
- Wear peaches paired with warm-toned shadows in brown, bronze, gold, and light or dark mossy green.
- Pink lips work with almost any eye color, as they duplicate the look of natural lips. Pink pairs especially well with grays and silver and navies.
- Nude tones are perfect for a no-makeup look or paired with bold eyes or smokey eyes in any shade.

LIP PRODUCTS

TINTED LIP BALM
Whether it's a stain or sheer lip balm, this is optimal for a nature-friendly look, days off, or while being active; often found with nourishing ingredients and SPF to protect aging lips. Tinted lip balm is a great buy, as they're rarely priced over $10.

LIP GLOSS
Glosses have different levels of viscosity from thin to thick—and come in endless shades. They can be layered over lipsticks for stronger staying power. Always use lip liner to help contain glosses in their borders and minimize bleeding. Lip glosses can intensify the sun's rays; always apply sunscreen on lips prior to use to prevent sun damage.

SHEER LIPSTICKS
These are the choice for natural lips. Usually very creamy in texture, they are significantly more transparent than cream lipsticks. The see-though consistency is a great choice for trying out new shades as they can be much more forgiving than full-coverage lip colors. Sheer lipsticks are the perfect alternative for mature lips, which may cause feathering from lip gloss. These lipsticks contain more moisturizing properties so they will deliver more shine, thereby creating a more youthful look. Plus, they're often found with antiaging properties, antioxidants, and sunscreen.

LIP CRAYON
Great for a quick lip application—and best of all, no mirrors are necessary. They're a must for busy multitaskers who need timesaving products. Lip crayons have the texture of a sheer lipstick without the need for a brush. They are found in an assortment of colors; you're bound to find one that's right for you!

CREAM LIPSTICKS
These offer intense pigment with light moisture and minimal shine. They're the ideal choice for mature lips that tend to bleed, or for those who need staying power. Cream lipsticks often come in long-wearing shades that last eight to sixteen hours and frequently have higher sun protection due to their opaque texture.

MATTE LIPSTICKS
Opaque and velvet in texture, matte colors are used often to achieve '30s to '50's looks, usually in orange or redder tones. The texture gives a more natural appearance to vibrant colors. In neutral or nude hues, matte lipsticks provide a '60s look. When coupled with a clean, natural eye, you can achieve a strong look using a bold color without too much makeup or effort. Matte lipsticks do contain minimal to no moisture, however, so if you have very dry lips opt for creamier textures.

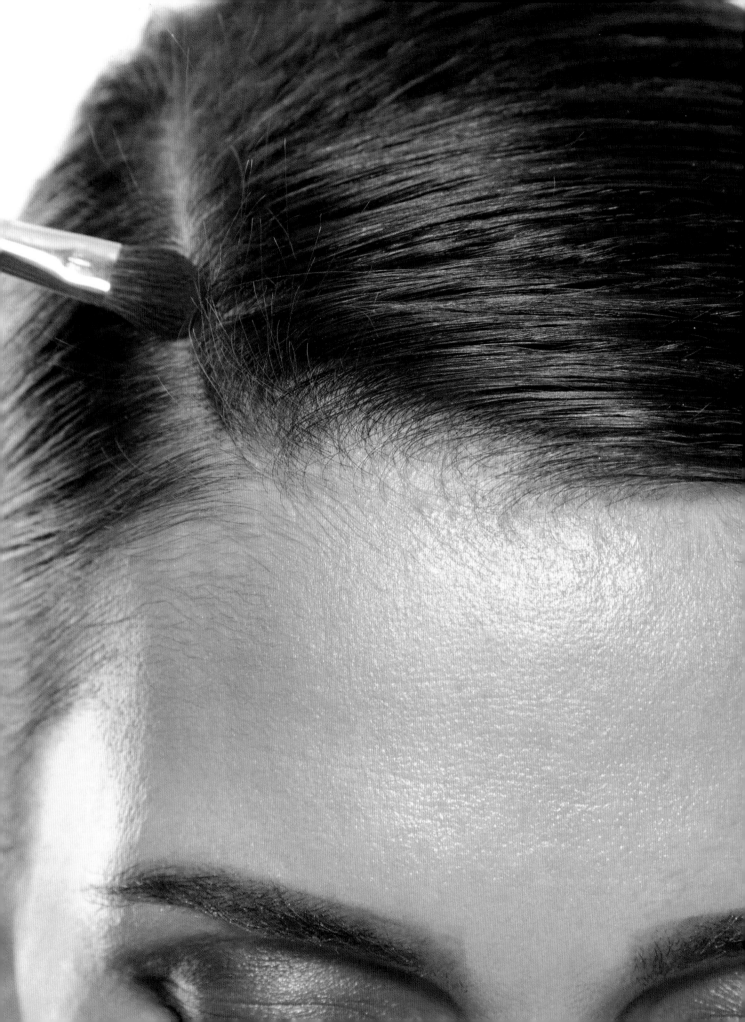

FAKING IT

Lifting the Veil on Red-Carpet Secrets

When I'm working as a makeup artist, I am likely hired to work on something special. It's not for selfies. It's usually because someone has to look her very best for a photo—generally for a magazine, to be on television, or on the coveted red carpet. It's essential that she looks like the best version of herself or she'll read about it. What most don't realize is the amount of work that goes into creating that look and into minimizing the look of aging. Even twenty-somethings get bronzer to create a youthful glow. Today, almost everyone is a celebrity. Your photos are ever more public thanks to friends tagging you in social media. It seems that all women are now in front of the camera, and the camera can often highlight the aging signs we hadn't seen before and freeze them in time. You don't have to look red-carpet ready at all times, but let's face it, it's the important days when we are supposed to look our very best that often make us feel the worst about ourselves. So be prepared. You'll be surprised how the extras make a big impact. It's actually simple extras that are essential to make your look go from good to great. It's the body glow, the bronzer, the filling in of the hairline, the shimmering legs that add the finishing touches to highlight your best assets.

HAIR

FOREHEAD LINES: BRONZER OR BANGS

Use bronzer on the temples and hairline to softly reline the hairline and give the area shape and dimension. This trick also minimizes a full forehead and adds a youthful glow to sallow skin.

You can never go wrong with bangs that drape across the forehead. Keep the swoop soft and touching the brows. This can require monthly maintenance (it also requires less Botox) and is a great way to add youthfulness and softness to the face. For longer bangs, swoop by the cheekbones and jawline to frame the face with softness.

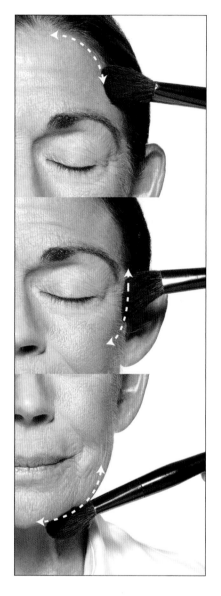

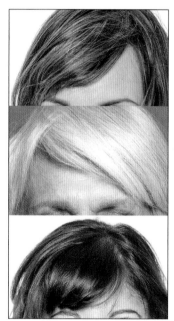

THE HAIRLINE

To create the illusion of a full hairline, make sure to keep your roots touched up. Faint, dull roots can make hair look even finer. Keep hairs looking full by making sure each strand is fully pigmented. You can fill in any sparse patches using an eye shadow brush and a dark shadow or brow powder to fill in above the temples and part, where hairs can be sparse and fine. This is especially important in the hairline part.

Over-the-counter hair fillers made of nylon fibers in various colors are also available at beauty supply stores. They attach to your skin and short hairs, and you can set with hairspray. They're a great way to fill in bald spots, especially close to the hairline and around the part, to give the illusion of fullness. Once the hairs are set, avoid touching them. Look for fibers that resemble the color of your hair that's close to your root. Use only the minimal amount of filler necessary; excessive amounts look less natural since no scalp shows through. If your hair color is between two different shades opt for the lighter-colored filler, to create a more natural look.

Take vitamins B and D, zinc, and iron to encourage healthy hair growth. Look for over-the-counter treatments that contain monoxodil, which can strengthen thinning hair and prevent future hair loss.

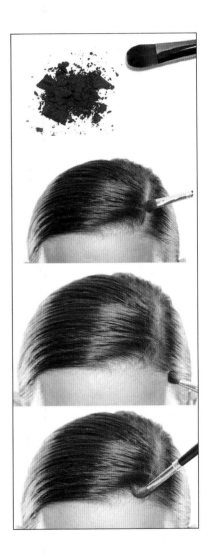

LEGS

One thing that has remained constant: Whether you're fifteen or fifty, anyone can use some help to make her legs look better. From moisturizers to bronzers or a little highlight on the front of your legs, leg makeup is something that everyone should learn to use. It can help make legs appear more toned and smooth.

To create the smoothest-looking legs:

1. Gently exfoliate legs using a loofah, salt, or sugar scrubs.
2. Moisturize legs, focusing on feet, knees, and ankles.
3. Apply self-tanner or temporary bronzing lotion using a bronzing mitt (preferable, as tanners will stain your hands), large brush, or your hands. Rub into skin using thin applications, making sure to blend in well. Wait for the first layer to dry before applying a second coat for a darker look. Make sure to wash your hands immediately after application to minimize staining.
4. If necessary, apply concealer to any veins visible after bronzer has been applied.
5. Finish with a shimmering highlight along the front of legs to create the illusion of length.

CHEST

One of the best and simplest ways to hide discoloration on your chest is to use foundation in your contour shade and blend it into your neck and chest area. This ensures that your face and chest area are uniform in color. Any differences in color will be obvious in photos; so be sure to fully blend in foundation if your chest is exposed when you're out on the town—in this era, everyone is a photographer!

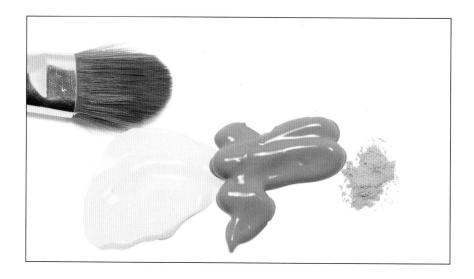

1. Make sure to moisturize neck and chest to ensure an even blend of foundation.
2. Apply a thin layer of foundation to your chest.
3. Tap on a second coat only where needed.
4. If necessary, apply concealer to any dark moles or spots.
5. Powder chest using a translucent powder with shimmer to help reflect discoloration.
6. Apply bronzer in the hollows of collarbone to add definition and on chest to add color.
7. Highlight the collarbones using a shimmer in opal or gold to accentuate and add dimension.

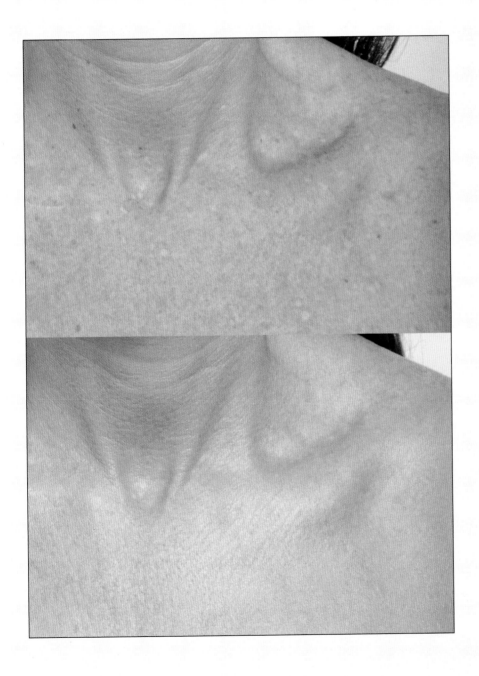

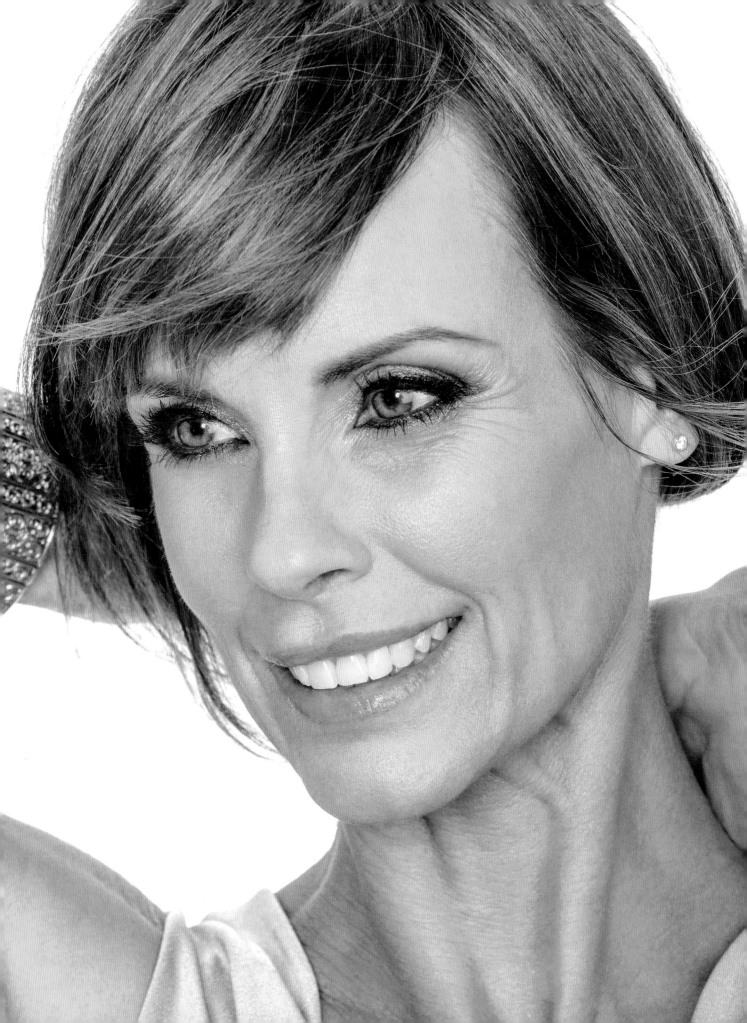

BEAUTY
BREAKDOWN

(arrows decorative)

THE NATURALIST

You pick up your skin-care products at the organic market. You examine the ingredients in your food and products to make sure that you are feeding your body and your skin as naturally as possible. Bar soap is not working like it used to, however, so you're thinking of taking things to the next level.

Skin care has changed dramatically and a lot of the products you are using are derived from fruits and their sugars. You can use homemade products to take care of your skin but they will not give you the results of cosmeceuticals, so it is essential that you take care of your skin through prevention. If you find yourself in the sun, make sure to wear loose, light clothing and use sunscreen and even use makeup to give yourself additional protection.

- Look for serums that are vitamin C based to rebuild collagen in the skin.
- Look for clay masks that contain sulfur and tea tree oil to purge impurities.
- Look for toners that have witch hazel to remove excess dirt.
- Look for exfoliants that contain alpha hydroxy acids to exfoliate skin.
- Look for sunscreens that contain titanium dioxide and micronized zinc oxide, which deliver sun protection without the white, pasty look.
- Eat good fats such as avocados, nuts, and olive oil.
- Incorporate strength training to naturally build human growth hormone (HGH).

THE PRODUCT JUNKIE

You want to look your best but want to stay away from the knife as long as possible, most likely forever. You're looking for the best skin care. You don't want to be the first for anything, and only use products and procedures that are tested and proven. You are curious about what will be the best minimally invasive cosmetic option for the best result. You look to makeup to create new, inspirational looks.

- Consult your dermatologist for the least invasive procedures and products. Try Retin-A for dull skin and products containing hydroquinone for sunspots before moving into more invasive processes. The earlier you start a preventive regimen, the better.
- In your forties and beyond, if skin is sagging significantly look to dermatological procedures such as resurfacing to renew the surface of the skin, and lifting procedures to help aggressively build new collagen.
- Make sure to strength train to build HGH, which will help your body repair itself and build collagen. Exercise also strengthens bones, which is essential to their health.
- Consume foods and vitamins that are high in antioxidants such as beans, dark green veggies including kale, and berries, to minimize cellular damage.
- Use masks that contain retinol to promote cell rejuvenation.
- Sunscreen is essential to minimize sun damage, especially if aggressive exfoliators are being used.

THE EARLY ADOPTER

A self-proclaimed skin expert, you are the first to try the newest products and latest in skin technologies, from skin-care products to procedures. You're on a first-name basis with your dermatologist and have a beauty team on speed dial for the latest and greatest. While you look to get the most bang for your buck, make sure to try a less invasive procedure prior to intensive treatments rather than leaping ahead. Take appropriate breaks in between procedures to allow your body to heal itself and get optimum results.

- Early adopters of skin treatments don't always wear much makeup. While skin treatment can help to lift and smooth the skin, it cannot replace the color loss that happens as we age. A little bit of color can brighten and help to create and finish the look you're trying to achieve. Something as simple as lining focal points like the eyes and lip line, and applying a hint of blush, can make all the difference.
- Make sure to use sunscreen to prevent sun damage, especially if you are exfoliating regularly and aggressively.
- Make sure to talk to your dermatologist if you use products that contain retinol or glycolic acid, which can affect procedures.
- Tell your doctor prior to procedures if you are taking any prescription or over-the-counter medications, including aspirin.

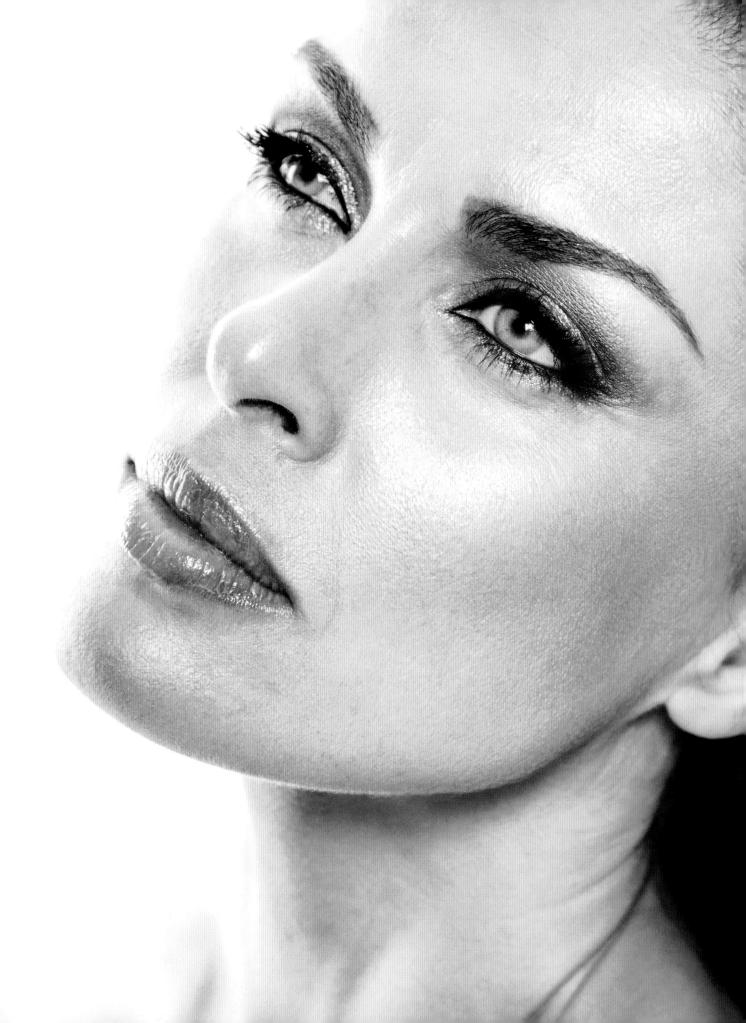

BEAUTY BY DECADE

HOW TO TAKE CARE OF AGING SKIN

There are common symptoms of aging that become more evident by the decade. Not everyone ages at the same pace, however. Some don't wrinkle at thirty; instead, their skin begins to hyperpigment and sag. Others get deeper lines in the forehead. Environment, genetics, and day-to-day beauty regimens play a big role in how we age. The following are common signs of aging as you move through each decade of life. If you have not started a beauty routine I urge you to begin with the simple skin-care regimen outlined in Chapter 1 before moving into more aggressive therapies. And remember to take care of yourself in the present; don't wait for a birthday or to lose ten pounds. You're beautiful now.

TWENTIES

PREVENTION

While your twenties are supposed to be carefree, how you take care of your skin during this time will be evident in your forties. Although the idea of thinking ahead this far can be daunting, believe me when I say it comes faster than you expect. And fine lines can come that much faster. Bad habits, like excessive caffeine, poor diet, smoking, sunbathing, and not removing makeup before bed can have lasting effects on your skin. If you haven't already, it's time to create strong beauty regimens that will last you a lifetime. Your skin's renewal is still working well, creating new skin pretty much on a monthly basis. Maintaining a strong skin-care routine and being consistent about damage prevention should be your main goals.

THIRTIES

CREATING SMOOTH SKIN

When you hit your thirties, your main concern will be fine lines, the beginnings of hyperpigmentation, and marionette lines, which occur as skin sags due to collagen breakdown. Make sure to pay attention to your chest area, as it is one of the most resilient in terms of skin cell regeneration. If you have not yet begun a skin-care regimen starting one now is essential. Skin turnover slows down in this decade; it's important to add serums into your routine, as their concentrated ingredients can encourage cell turnover. Begin using masks, which promote cellular turnover and infuse moisture and vitamins into the skin, once a week.

FORTIES

SPOT-FREE SKIN

Moving into perimenopause, skin begins to thin as fat loss in the face increases. Quality of sleep can start to decrease. Hair becomes thinner on the scalp as well as in brows and eyelashes. It's essential to take care of your nutrition during this time and exercise to mitigate stress. There are often two very different types of aging that happen during these times. Some women will tend to develop deeper wrinkles while others experience dark spots and sagging. Use appropriate products with more aggressive exfoliation to reduce surface dryness and wrinkles as well as minimize spots. Products with hydroquinone or retinol can help to minimize spotting. And be sure to use sunscreen, especially when exfoliating. Be diligent about your morning and evening skin-care routines and talk to your dermatologist if you are looking for more aggressive treatments.

FIFTIES

DEFYING GRAVITY AND ADDING COLOR

Skin is very much affected by hormones. Often referred to as the desert decade, your fifties is a period when skin loses a lot of its moisture as well as fullness, which can cause additional sagging. Skin is more stressed. Menopause is a factor and hormones need to be considered. Make sure to talk to your doctor about caring for the inside as well as the outside, as hormones can cause changes in your body as well as in your mood.

SIXTIES AND BEYOND

FOCUSING ON DEFINITION

As skin loses pigment as well as facial hairs, the lines that define features fade drastically. Focus on makeup products that deliver big returns in little time, like eyebrow color, eyeliner, and lipstick to enhance features.

Thirtysomething

NAME: Marcela Isaza

AGE: 36

OCCUPATION: Red Carpet reporter

DESCRIBE YOURSELF: I am a bilingual entertainment TV reporter and have interviewed Oprah, Angelina Jolie, Tom Cruise, Jennifer Lopez, Juanes, and tons of other superstars. I am a Colombian-born, L.A.-raised chica, so basically it's in my DNA to care about antiaging, ha! Plus I'm pretty witty, a bit quirky, and almost always try to remain very enthusiastic about life.

I AM INSPIRED BY: People who have overcome the impossible, make it big, then turn around, and give it all back, for example, Oprah Winfrey.

I AM HAPPIEST WHEN: While I get to sit face-to-face daily with A-list Hollywood stars, my favorite part of the day is coming home to hear how my daughter's day at school was. She truly is my sunshine.

I FEEL MY BEST WHEN: I take time to love and respect myself. I do this by eating healthy, exercising regularly, allowing myself a good night's rest, finding joy in life's simple blessings, and laughing as much as I can. A large glass of wine helps, too . . .

MY BEAUTY ICON: Cindy Crawford and Christy Turlington. I was a teenager in the '90s when billboards featured supermodels, not celebrities.

I CAN'T LIVE WITHOUT: I can't live without laughter. A smile and a good laugh can cure anything. I also can't live without having faith. Faith doesn't make things easy, it makes them possible.

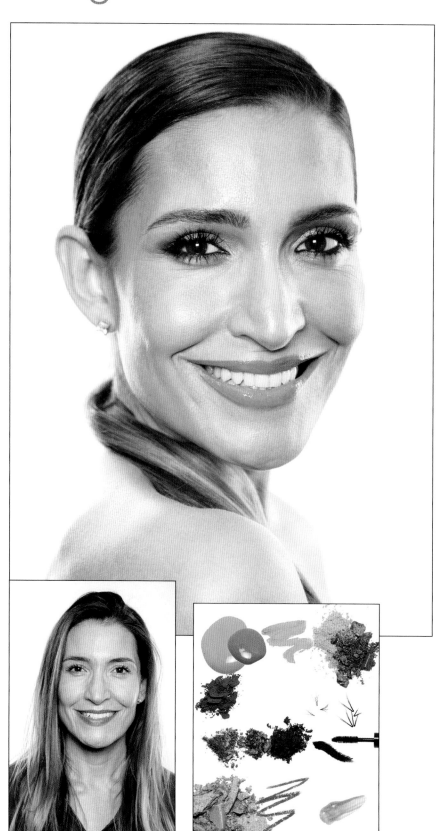

SKIN

1. Apply golden-beige foundation all over the face and neck.
2. Contour using tan fluid foundation to the outside edges of the face, the temples, the cheeks, sides of the nose, and under the jawline.
3. Apply a beige concealer under the eyes.
4. Set foundation using a sheer yellow loose powder.
5. Apply bronzer along the cheekbones and temples.
6. Apply shimmering blush at the apples of the cheeks and under the jawline.

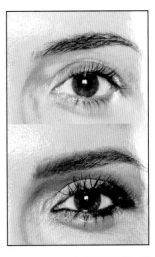

EYES

1. Apply dark gold eye shadow to the base of the lids.
2. Apply bronze eye shadow to the outside corners of the eyes and slightly above the creases.
3. Apply espresso eye shadow to the outside corners of the eyes to add depth.
4. Apply dark brown eyeliner along the top of the lash lines and extend at a 45-degree angle slightly to the outside corners of the eyes.

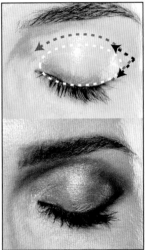

LASHES

1. Curl eyelashes at the base, middle, and tips.
2. Apply two coats of volumizing mascara to the top and bottom lashes.
3. Apply V-shaped individual black false eyelashes sporadically along the lash lines and fill with individual short lashes.

BROWS

1. Apply medium-brown powder along the top of brows and lightly fill in the sparse areas and the tails of the brows.

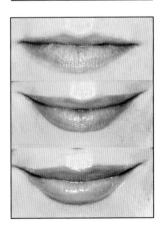

LIPS

1. Apply medium-brown lip liner slightly above the natural lip line and lightly fill in lips.
2. Apply peach lip gloss to the entire mouth over the natural lip line.

Fabulous Forties

NAME: Wendy Both

AGE: 41

OCCUPATION: Model, Reiki Master

DESCRIBE YOURSELF: I was born in Holland, to a Dutch mother and Indian/Indonesian father, and now live in Los Angeles with my daughter. My huge bucket list contains world travel and adventure. I am a Reiki master and teacher and treat both people and animals. I cherish my large group of friends, and laughter is never absent. I am a bit of an adrenaline junkie, and Motocross is one such activity I enjoy tremendously. I continuously increase my knowledge on mental health disorders and metaphysical and spiritual subjects. My biggest accomplishment in life is my sweet daughter.

I AM INSPIRED BY: My sweet daughter. Unconditional love. Baring one's soul for self-growth. Courage.

WHAT BRINGS YOU JOY: My daughter. Beauty of nature. Animals. Laughing. Desire to help others on their healing path. Listening to Reggae Music.

I FEEL MY BEST WHEN: I eat healthy.

MY BEAUTY ICON: Sophia Loren.

I CAN'T LIVE WITHOUT: A cup of coffee in the morning.

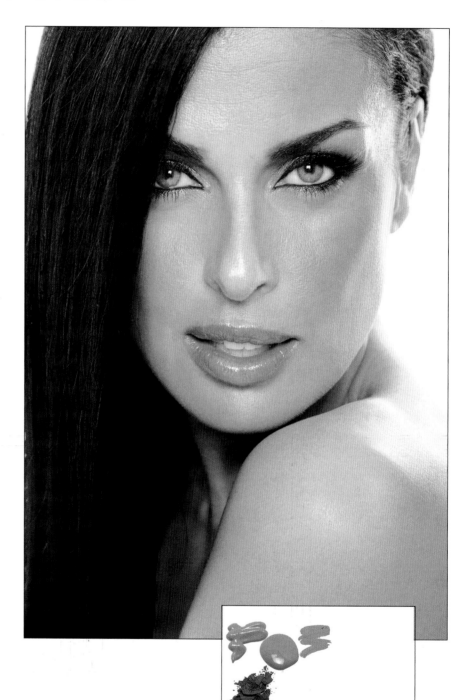

SKIN

1. Apply warm beige cream foundation all over the face and neck.
2. Contour using a tan fluid foundation to the outside edges of the face, the temples, the cheeks, sides of the nose, and under the jawline.
3. Apply ocher concealer under the eyes.
4. Apply a shimmering peach blush at the apples of the cheeks.

EYES

1. Apply dark gold eye shadow to the base of the lid, along the lower lash lines and at the inner corners.
2. Apply olive-green eye shadow to the outside top and bottom corners of the eyes.
3. Apply black eye shadow to the outside top and bottom corners of the eyes.
4. Apply black cream eyeliner along the top of the lash lines and at a 45-degree angle at the outside corners of the eyes.
5. Apply black pencil liner inside the waterline to add intensity to the eyes.

LASHES

1. Curl eyelashes at the base and middle.
2. Apply two coats of volumizing mascara to the top and bottom lashes.
3. Apply corner black false eyelashes to the outside corners of the eyes.

BROWS

1. Apply medium-brown brow powder, lightly filling in the sparse areas.
2. Apply a dark brown brow powder to the tails of the brows.

LIPS

1. Apply soft brown lip liner slightly above the natural lip line.
2. Apply sheer nude lip gloss over the entire mouth.

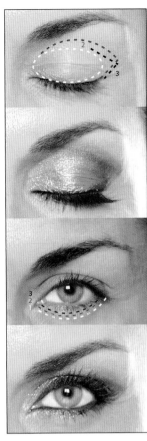

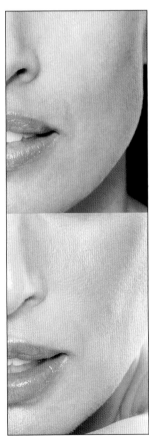

The New Fifty: Getting Glam

NAME: Valerie Van Galder

AGE: 51, and I have never felt better!

OCCUPATION: Marketing executive

DESCRIBE YOURSELF: A serial monogamist in all things craft, including but not limited to: knitting, crochet, embroidery, painting, and quilting. Currently obsessed with becoming a world-class cake designer. Have run marathons and may run more. A wife, a daughter, an aunt, a stepmom, and a sister. About to make a huge career change, going to work for the Walt Disney Imagineers, which is the fulfillment of a lifelong dream.

I AM INSPIRED BY: People who use their powers for good.

WHAT BRINGS YOU JOY: Too many things to list. As I type this, my dog is curled on my lap. That is certainly one of them.

I FEEL MY BEST WHEN: I am feeding the people whom I love the food I have cooked for them.

MY BEAUTY ICON: Edie Sedgwick.

I CAN'T GO WITHOUT: My weekly trip to the blow-dry bar.

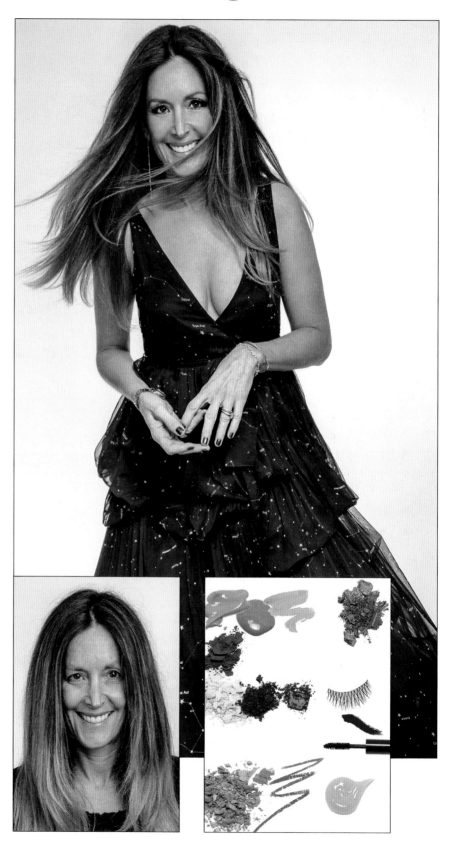

SKIN

1. Apply a beige cream foundation all over the face and neck.
2. Contour using a tan cream foundation to the outside edges of the face, the temples, the cheeks, sides of the nose, and under the jawline.
3. Apply beige concealer under the eyes.
4. Set foundation using a translucent loose powder.
5. Apply bronzer along the cheekbones and temples.
6. Apply pink shimmering blush at the apples of the cheeks.

EYES

1. Apply shimmering opal eye shadow base to the base of the lids and along the bottom lash lines and inner corners.
2. Apply dark brown contour eye shadow to the outside corners of the eyes in a horizontal V shape under the brow bone and above the crease.
3. Apply a navy blue eye shadow along and close to the lash lines, applying up at a 45-degree angle.
4. Apply black eyeliner along the top and bottom lash lines at a 45-degree angle to extend the outside corners of the eyes. Apply in the waterline to create a smokey, sultry effect.

LASHES

1. Curl eyelashes at the base, middle, and tips.
2. Apply two coats of black mascara to the top and bottom lashes.
3. Apply strip eyelashes to open and add drama to the eyes.

BROWS

1. Apply light brown brow powder along the tops of brows and lightly fill in the entire brow using short, hairlike strokes, then extend the tails of the brows.

LIPS

1. Apply nude lip liner slightly above the natural lip line.
2. Apply sheer pinky-beige lipstick on the entire mouth covering the lip liner.
3. Apply a shimmering beige lip gloss to the center of the mouth.

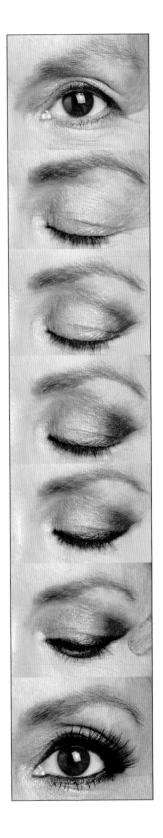

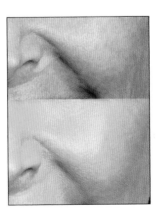

Enchanting Sixties

NAME: Maye Musk

AGE: 66

OCCUPATION: Model/ Nutritionist

DESCRIBE YOURSELF: I'm a nerd; I love science and math. I spend most of my time reading nutrition research, counseling clients, giving presentations, and consulting to the food and health industry. My other work is modeling, which has become busier as I've gotten older. Who knew? I travel a lot for both careers and enjoy learning about different cultures. The rest of my time is spent with my three kids, ten grandchildren, and large family, which brings me great joy.

I AM INSPIRED BY: I am easily inspired by everyone and everything I see and learn about every day. I wake up with a positive attitude and with a lot of energy. I love my work, whether as a dietician or a model, and get down to business right away. I have tried to help negative people in the past, but found they actually don't want to change. Now I mix only with happy, considerate, kind, creative, and intelligent people.

WHAT BRINGS YOU JOY: My kids, grandchildren, huge family, dog, friends, nutrition work, modeling, and traveling.

I FEEL MY BEST WHEN: I'm eating well, working out, and enjoying good health. I love to dress well and look great when going out.

MY BEAUTY ICON: My late mother, who never knew she was beautiful as no one told her until she was in her eighties. She was natural, charming, and kind to everyone. Thank you for giving me your cheekbones, Mom!

I CAN'T LIVE WITHOUT: Food, but I think you mean beauty-wise. For that, I can't go without lip balm.

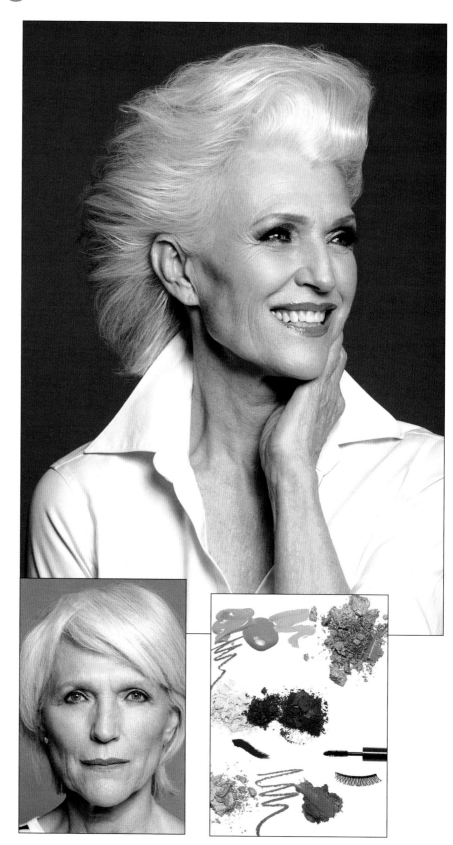

SKIN

1. Apply a beige cream foundation all over the face and neck. Apply a second layer over the cheeks and nose area for extra coverage.
2. Contour using a tan fluid foundation to the outside edges of the face, the temples, the cheekbones, sides of the nose, and under the jawline.
3. Set foundation using translucent loose powder.
4. Apply medium-brown bronzer along the cheekbones and temples.
5. Apply a shimmering pink blush at the apples of the cheeks.

EYES

1. Apply opal eye shadow to the base of the lids and along the bottom lash line.
2. Apply dark brown eye shadow to the outside corners of the eyes and above the crease.
3. Apply black eye shadow to the outside corners of the eyes and above the crease.
4. Apply opal eye shadow to the inside corners of the eyes.
5. Apply dark brown eye shadow along the lower lash line.
6. Apply black cream eyeliner along the top of the lash line and angle at a 45-degree angle and along the lower lash lines.

LASHES

1. Curl eyelashes at the base and middle.
2. Apply two coats of waterproof volumizing mascara to the top and bottom lashes.
3. Apply a full strip of soft-volume black false eyelashes to the eyes.

BROWS

1. Apply ash-brown brow pencil along the top of brows to create a higher arch. Extend and darken the tails and lightly fill in the brows using short, hairlike strokes.

LIPS

1. Apply warm-brown lip liner slightly above the natural lip line and fill in.
2. Apply a creamy raspberry lipstick on the entire mouth, covering the lip liner.

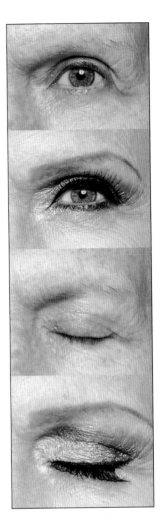

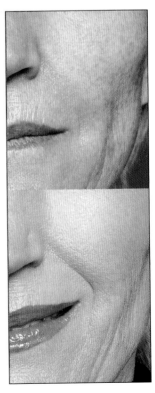

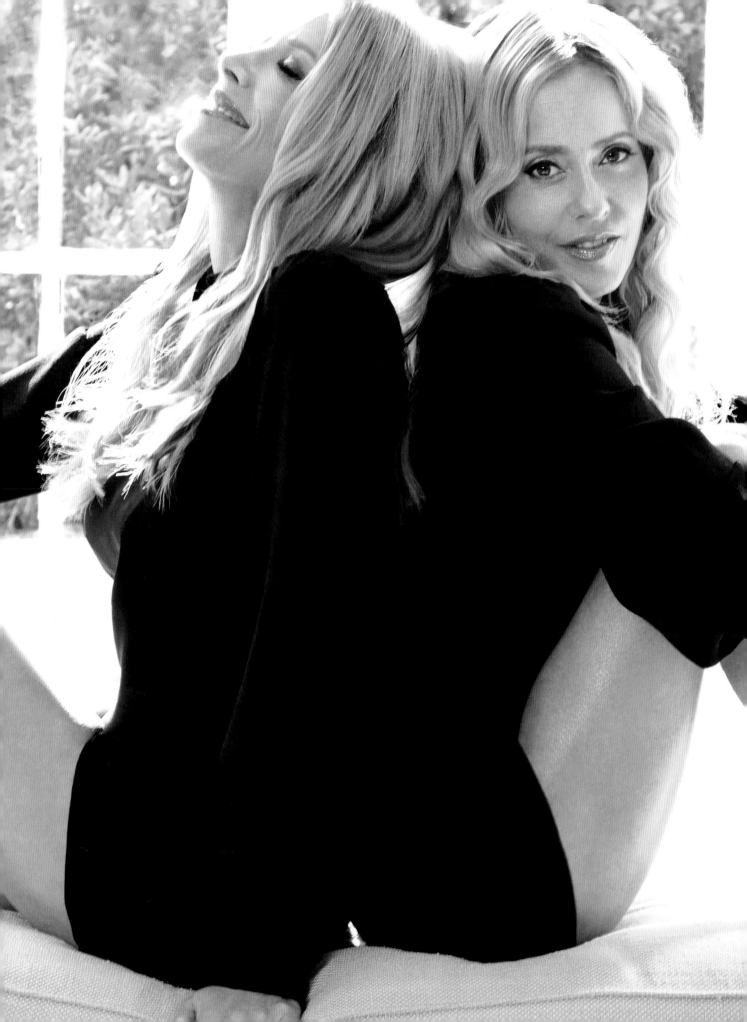

BEAUTY EVOLUTION

Creating Your Own Beauty

I've always loved makeovers. Seeing the look on a woman's face after I've applied just a few products and then watching her face light up makes the hairs on my arms stand up. Even today, after having performed thousands of them, there's a connection that happens. A woman sees herself almost for the first time as she really is. I never understood why women felt bad about getting makeovers because my connection to them was so positive. And then I looked up the word in the dictionary.

make·o·ver [meyk-oh-ver] noun
1. Remodeling; renovation; restoration
2. A thorough course of beauty and cosmetic treatments

Just reading the definition sounds exhausting. And I realized this is how other people perceive a makeover. It implies an overhaul, too, often in the vision of the artist but without consideration of the person, the event, and most important their comfort level. And that has never been my intention when I work with someone. It's always been about showing someone how to create their own beauty.

Creating your beauty when aging is more of an evolution of yourself, not a redo; after all, there is a comfort in knowing your likes and dislikes. Any changes you make should help define who you are and who you want to become.

Every morning is an opportunity for you to create your own beauty and show the world who you are. As you age and get to know yourself a little better more and more each day, this look will continue to evolve. The way you look should always reflect how you want to be perceived. It should empower you to better take on your day, whether it's in a courtroom or a playground, and whether you are twenty-five or eighty-five. The best part is that you can create different looks for the different aspects of your life or your mood—because we are more than our job or our titles. Try multiple makeup looks to see which makes you feel your best you.

BEFORE

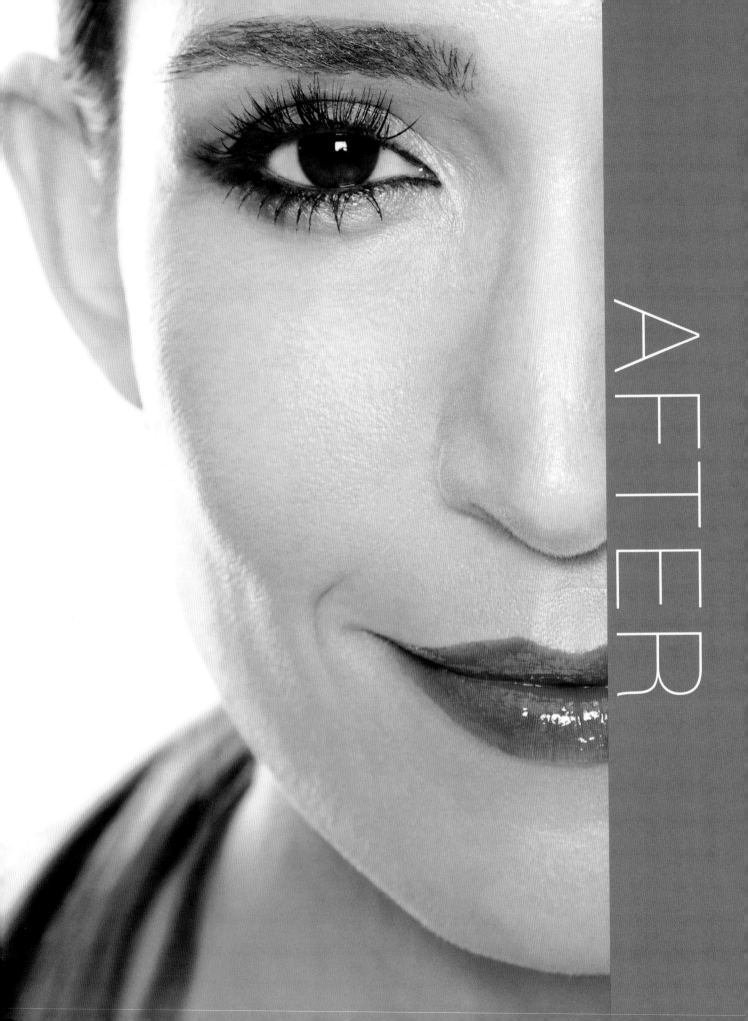

AFTER

Global Glamour

KELI LEE

AGE: 42

OCCUPATION: Casting Executive

DESCRIBE YOURSELF:
Multitasker, world traveler, speaker, lover of giving back, fashion, and great food. I run casting for ABC Television Network and ABC Studios and search the globe for talent.

I AM INSPIRED BY: Traveling to new places, meeting new people, and learning about different cultures. I'm also inspired by my friends, by imperfection, and those who have overcome adversity and achieved success.

I AM HAPPIEST WHEN: I'm surrounded by my friends and family and when I have high-speed Wi-Fi and the Internet, with multiple-device connectivity.

I FEEL MY BEST WHEN: I'm eating healthy and being active and outdoors.

MY BEAUTY ICON: Julianne Moore. She is beautiful and graceful without plastic surgery.

I CAN'T LIVE WITHOUT: Friends and family, traveling the world, high-speed Wi-Fi, my iPhone and iPad and their chargers, mascara, eyeliner, and eyelash curler!

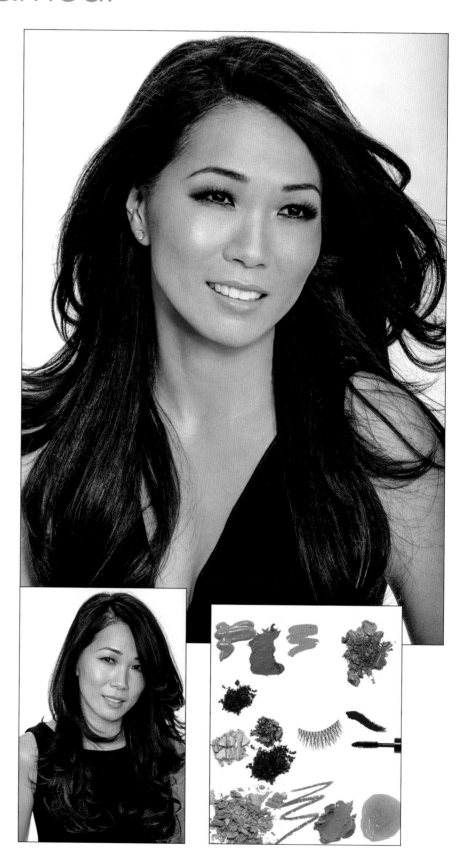

SKIN

1. Apply warm beige cream foundation to the center of the face, eyelids, under eyes, bridge of nose, and the chin.
2. Contour using a chestnut-brown cream foundation to the outside edges of the face, the temples, the cheeks, sides of the nose and under the jawline and hairline to add depth.
3. Apply medium-bronze bronzer along the cheekbones and temples.
4. Apply pale pink blush at the apples of the cheeks.

EYES

1. Apply pale gold eye shadow to the base of the lids and along the bottom lash lines, extending at the outside corners.
2. Layer dark bronze eye shadow to the base of the lids and along the bottom lash lines, extending at the outside corners.
3. Apply dark brown matte eye shadow from lash lines to slightly above the creases and along the outside lower lash lines.
4. Apply black cream eyeliner around the entire eyes, smudging slightly.
5. Apply pale gold highlighting eye shadow to the inside corners of the eyes.

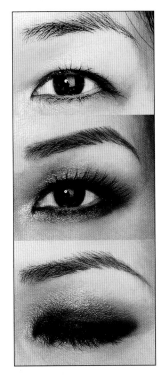

LASHES

1. Curl eyelashes at the base, middle, and tips.
2. Apply two coats of waterproof volumizing black mascara to the top and bottom lashes.
3. Apply full-length-strip eyelashes.

BROWS

1. Apply medium-ash-brown brow powder along the tops of brows and lightly fill in the sparse areas. Fill in the tails of the brows.

LIPS

1. Apply natural lip liner slightly above the natural lip line.
2. Apply a beige lipstick on the entire mouth, covering the lip liner.
3. Apply a shimmering sheer peach lip gloss over the entire mouth.

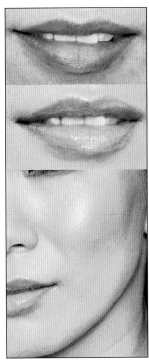

Fearless in Fashion

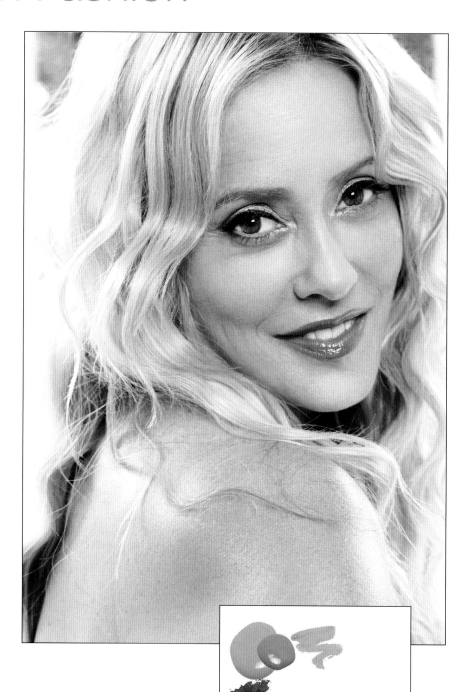

NAME: Pamela Skaist-Levy

AGE: 50

OCCUPATION: Fashion designer

DESCRIBE YOURSELF: Mother, wife, fashion designer, surf rat, Etsy addict, f**king great friend, and obsessed with Joni Mitchell.

I AM INSPIRED BY: All things good and beautiful.

I AM HAPPIEST WHEN: I'm in nature with my family, when I'm totally present. In my youth when I was at work I was feeling guilty about not being with my son, and when I was with my son I was feeling guilty about not being at work. I now live in the moment and that makes for a balanced, happy life.

MY BEAUTY ICON: Joni Mitchell. Not only do I love her look and vibe, her music takes her to another level in terms of beauty and style.

I CAN'T LIVE WITHOUT: The perfume Carnal Flower by Frederic Malle. The tuberose blossoms exude pure happiness.

SKIN

1. Apply a sheer beige fluid foundation all over the face and neck.
2. Contour using a sheer tan foundation to the outside edges of the face, the temples, the cheeks, sides of the nose, and under the jawline.
3. Apply beige concealer under the eyes.
4. Set foundation using a translucent loose powder.
5. Apply golden-bronze bronzer along the cheekbones, temples, and hairline.
6. Apply pink blush at the apples of the cheeks.

EYES

1. Apply shimmering opal eye shadow to the base of the lids and along the bottom lash lines and inner corners.
2. Apply dark-ash-brown contour eye shadow to the outside corners of the eyes.
3. Apply black eyeliner along the top of the lash lines and angle upward at a 45-degree angle at the outside corners of the eyes, extending farther than the lash line.

LASHES

1. Curl eyelashes at the base, middle, and tips.
2. Apply two coats of black mascara to the top and bottom lashes.
3. Apply corner half lashes to the outside corners of the eyes.

BROWS

1. Apply light brown brow powder along the tops of brows and lightly fill in, extending down the tails of the brows.

LIPS

1. Apply nude lip liner slightly above the natural lip line.
2. Apply coral-red lipstick to the entire mouth, covering the lip liner.

Cali-Centric Glamour

NAME: Gela Nash Taylor

OCCUPATION: Designer

DESCRIBE YOURSELF: I am a mother, a wife, and a major workaholic . . . obsessed with fashion, and a makeup/product junkie!

I AM INSPIRED BY: The nature that surrounds me . . . light and color.

WHAT BRINGS YOU JOY: My family and friends bring me endless joy as does my work!

I FEEL MY BEST WHEN: I am happy and productive . . . and smothered in Carnal Flower.

MY BEAUTY ICON: Georgiana Duchess of Devonshire, and who isn't obsessed with Kate and Twiggy?

I CAN'T GO WITHOUT: Moisturizer . . . and gallons of water.

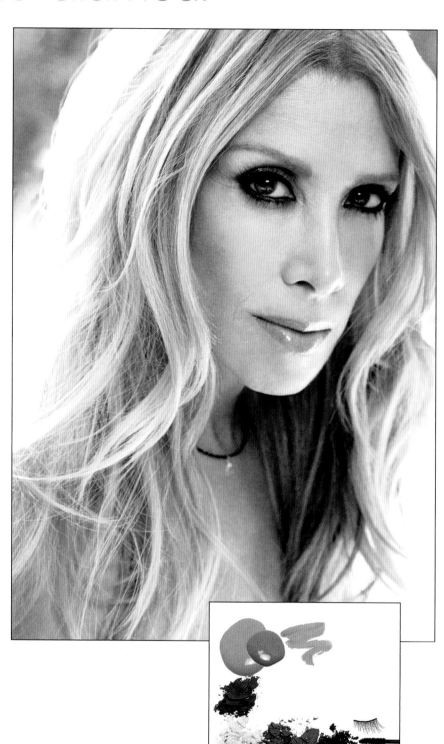

SKIN

1. Apply a beige fluid foundation all over the face and neck.
2. Contour using a medium-brown fluid foundation to the outside edges of the face, the temples, the cheeks, sides of the nose, and under the jawline.
3. Apply beige concealer under the eyes.
4. Apply medium-ash bronzer along the cheekbones and temples.
5. Apply pale pink blush at the apples of the cheeks.

EYES

1. Apply plum eyeshadow to the base of and along the bottom lash line.
2. Apply shimmering opal eye shadow to the center of the base of the lids, under lash lines, and on the inner corners of the eyes.
3. Apply dark brown eye shadow to the outside top and bottom corners of the eyes.
4. Apply black cream eyeliner along the top of the lash lines and at a 45-degree angle at the outside corners of the eyes.
5. Apply black waterproof eyeliner to the inside waterline.

LASHES

1. Curl eyelashes at the base, middle, and tips.
2. Apply two coats of volumizing mascara to the top and bottom lashes.
3. Apply half or corner black false eyelashes to the outside corners of the eyes.

BROWS

1. Apply ash-brown brow powder along the tops of brows and lightly fill in and extend the tails of the brows.

LIPS

1. Apply nude lip liner slightly above the natural lip line.
2. Apply a pale peachy-nude lipstick to the entire mouth, covering the lip liner.
3. Apply clear lip gloss to the center of the mouth.

Red-Carpet Ready

NAME: Jes Macallan

AGE: Well . . . I feel 21 in party time; 31 in real time; and 51 in life-experience time!

OCCUPATION: Actress

DESCRIBE YOURSELF: I grew up a dancer, transitioned into acting, and am very passionate about my work. I am *enamored* by people. I am also a humanitarian at the core and am a bleeding heart. I constantly want to learn about people and their pasts. I especially love the elderly. I could listen to stories of love, and life, and loss forever.

I AM INSPIRED BY: Passion, originality, and people who have a different perspective on things. I think the people I am always attracted to seem to have one or more of these.

I AM HAPPIEST WHEN: Feeling challenged in an intelligent way invigorates me and brings me joy. I love debates. I love a good competitive game night filled with friends and laughter and wine! I love my gigantic family, complete with six brothers and sisters. I love my husband and all of my crazy animals . . .

I FEEL MY BEST WHEN: I challenge myself to go after something that I know I want but I am avoiding, or fighting, or putting off because of insecurities, fear, etc. When I finally just do it—even if it is just some silly cooking class or something more monumental like writing that passion-piece script I can't stop thinking about—I feel my best that I went and did it.

MY BEAUTY ICON: Lucille Ball

I CAN'T LIVE WITHOUT: Oxygen (obvious) or . . . *love* . . . which I think is an even more obvious answer.

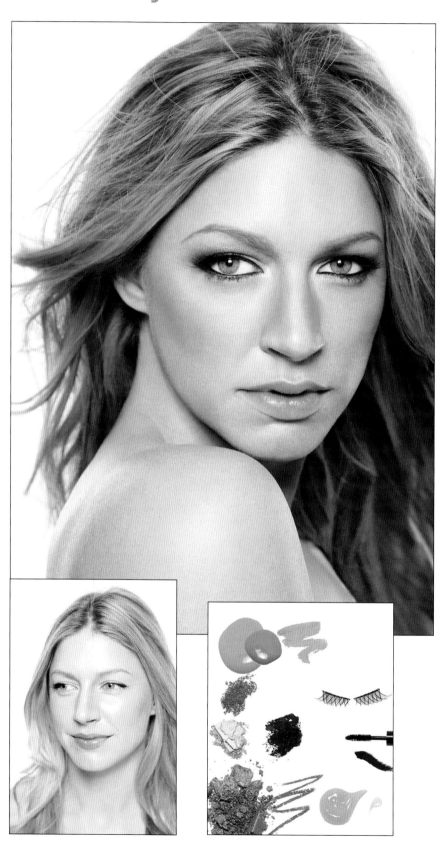

SKIN

1. Apply a warm beige fluid foundation all over the face and neck.
2. Contour using a tan fluid foundation to the outside edges of the face, the temples, the cheekbones, sides of the nose, and under the jawline.
3. Set foundation using a translucent loose powder.
4. Apply golden bronzer along the cheekbones, temples, and hairline to create a bronzed look.
5. Apply golden bronzer lightly to the apples of the cheeks to add warmth.

EYES

1. Apply pale silver eye shadow to the base of the inner corners of the lids and along the bottom lash line.
2. Apply black eye shadow to the outside corners of the eyes, angling the outside corners up above the entire crease to create a slightly rounded shape.
3. Apply black eye shadow along the lower lash line.
4. Apply black cream eyeliner along the top of the lash lines at a 45-degree angle at the outside corners of the eyes.
5. Apply black waterproof pencil eyeliner inside the waterline.

LASHES

1. Curl eyelashes at the base, middle, and tips.
2. Apply two coats of volumizing mascara to the top and bottom lashes.
3. Apply long corner black false eyelashes to the outside corners of the eyes.

BROWS

1. Apply light-ash-brown brow powder to fill in the beginning of the brows and along the tops of brows, and lightly fill in the sparse areas.
2. Apply a medium-ash-brown to the tails of the brows.

LIPS

1. Apply nude lip liner slightly above the natural lip line and lightly fill in.
2. Apply sheer pinky-nude lip balm over the entire lip.
3. Apply clear gloss to the entire mouth.

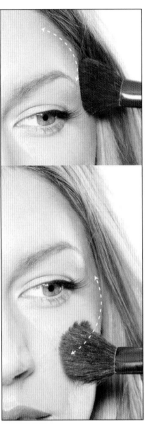

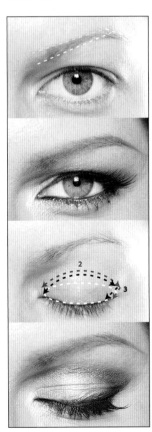

Strong and Smokey

NAME: Stephanie Liner

AGE: 48

OCCUPATION: Real estate developer/designer

DESCRIBE YOURSELF: Mommy, wife, friend, stubborn type A, lover of beauty . . . interior design, Paris, architecture. I'm trying to make a difference on this planet in some small way.

WHAT INSPIRES YOU? To see people happy from my work. My children inspire me to be a better person and to always try to do the "right" thing. And, Paris.

WHAT BRINGS YOU JOY: Hearing my kids call me "Mommy" . . . even as they get older. My little dog Nelson. The love I get and feel from my husband.

I FEEL BEST WHEN: I take the time to take care of myself. Eating well. When I am working. When I am relaxing with my family.

MY BEAUTY ICON: Grace Kelly and Jackie Onassis.

I CAN'T LIVE WITHOUT: Paris.

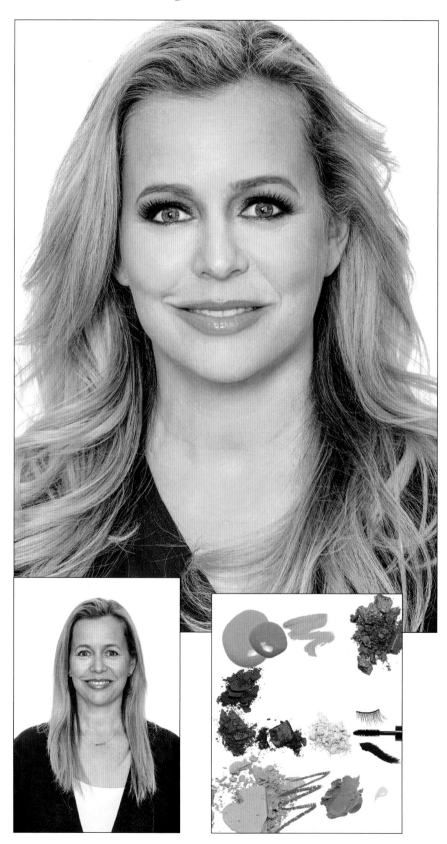

SKIN

1. Apply a warm beige foundation all over the face and neck.
2. Contour using tan fluid foundation to the outside edges of the face, the temples, the cheeks, sides of the nose, and under the jawline.
3. Set foundation using translucent loose powder.
4. Apply bronzer along the cheekbones and temples, under the jawline, and along the hairline.
5. Apply pale pink blush at the apples of the cheeks.

EYES

1. Apply shimmering plum eye shadow to the base of the lids.
2. Apply eggplant eye shadow to the outside corners of the eyes and blend, applying slightly above the crease.
3. Apply black cream eyeliner along the tops of the lash lines at a 45-degree angle at the outside corners of the eyes.
4. Blend eyeliner using eggplant eye shadow along the top lash lines to create softer, smokey eyes.
5. Apply black pencil eyeliner inside the waterline.

LASHES

1. Curl eyelashes at the base, middle, and tips.
2. Apply two coats of volumizing mascara to the top and bottom lashes.
3. Apply a full-strip false eyelashes strip with crisscrossing varying lengths to the lash line.

BROWS

1. Apply light-ash-brown brow powder along the top of brows and lightly fill in the sparse areas and above the arch. Extend the tails of the brows.

LIPS

1. Apply nude lip liner slightly above the natural lip line.
2. Apply nude cream lipstick on the entire mouth covering the lip liner.
3. Apply clear lip gloss to the center of the mouth.

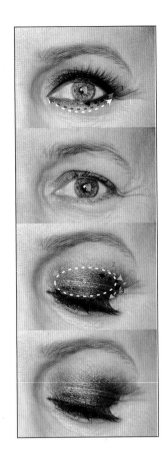

Beautiful and Brilliant

NAME: Jackie Barton

AGE: 61

OCCUPATION: Scientist

DESCRIBE YOURSELF: Wife, mom, and scientist.

WHAT INSPIRES YOU? Chemistry, the research with my students, and learning more about how the world works.

WHAT BRINGS YOU JOY? Spending time with my daughter, Elizabeth.

I FEEL MY BEST WHEN: I'm sitting on the porch with my husband, Peter, looking over the ocean in Laguna.

MY BEAUTY ICON: Audrey Hepburn.

I CAN'T LIVE WITHOUT: My Christian Louboutin high heels!

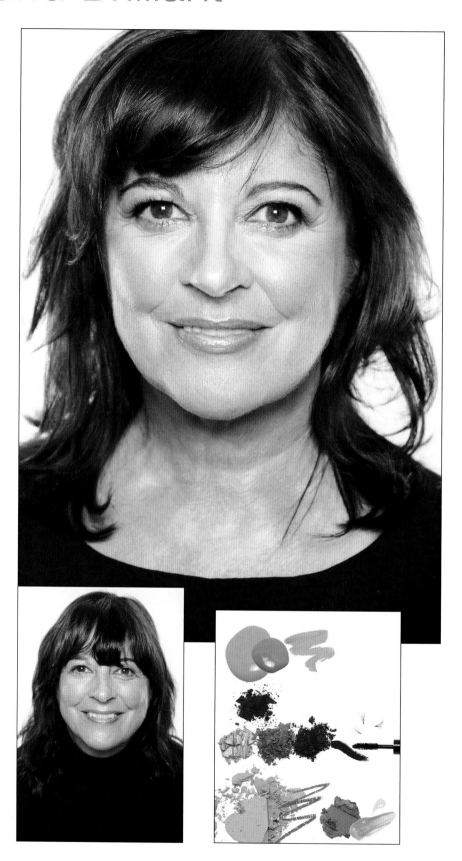

SKIN

1. Apply medium beige foundation all over the face and neck.
2. Contour using a tan foundation to the outside edges of the face, the temples, the cheeks, sides of the nose, and under the jawline.
3. Apply pale blush at the apples of the cheeks.

EYES

1. Apply pale gold eye shadow to the base of the lids and along the bottom lash lines.
2. Apply warm taupe eye shadow to the outside corners of the eyes and above the crease, to create a slightly round shape.
3. Apply dark brown eye shadow to the outside corners of the eyes and along the outside corners of the bottom lash lines.
4. Apply pale gold eye shadow to the inside corners of the eyes.
5. Apply black cream eyeliner along the top of the lash lines and at a 45-degree angle at the outside corners of the eyes.

LASHES

1. Curl eyelashes at the base and middle.
2. Apply two coats of mascara to the top and bottom lashes.
3. Apply individual short black false eyelashes to the outside corners of the eyes.

BROWS

1. Apply medium-brown eyebrow powder along the tops of brows and lightly fill in the top of the arch to create a slightly higher brow. Apply to the tails of the brows.

LIPS

1. Apply medium-brown lip liner slightly above the natural lip line.
2. Apply warm apricot lipstick to the entire mouth, covering the lip liner.
3. Apply shimmering peach lip gloss to the center of the mouth.

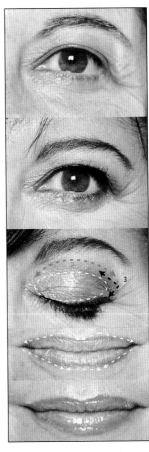

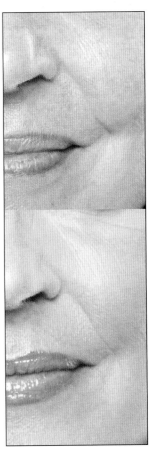

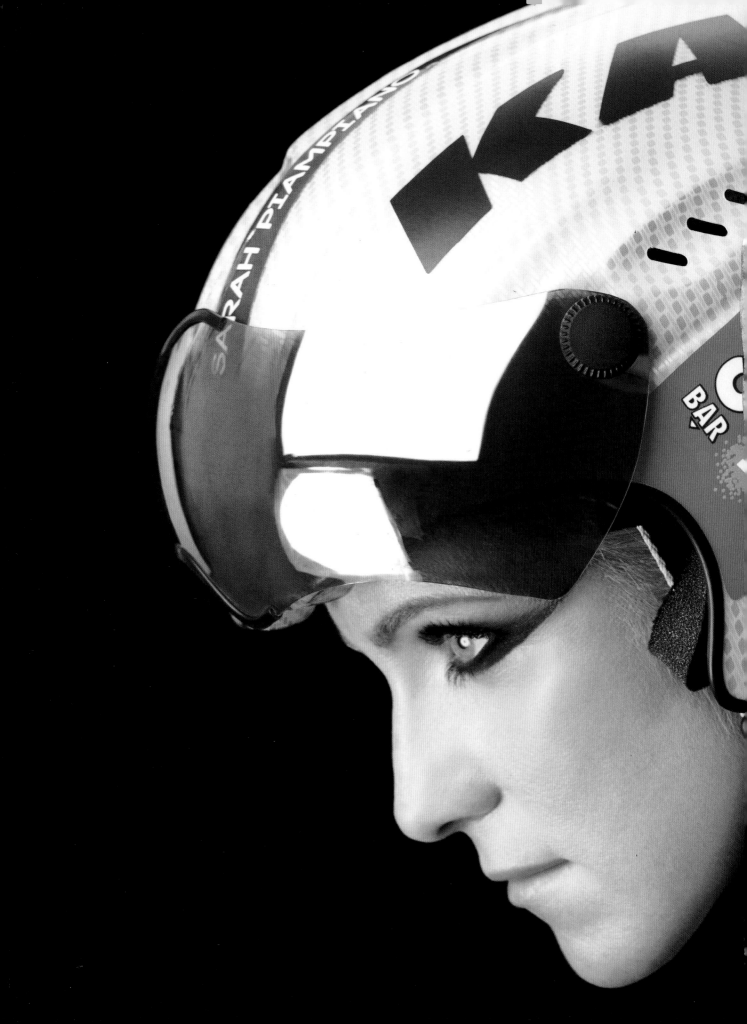

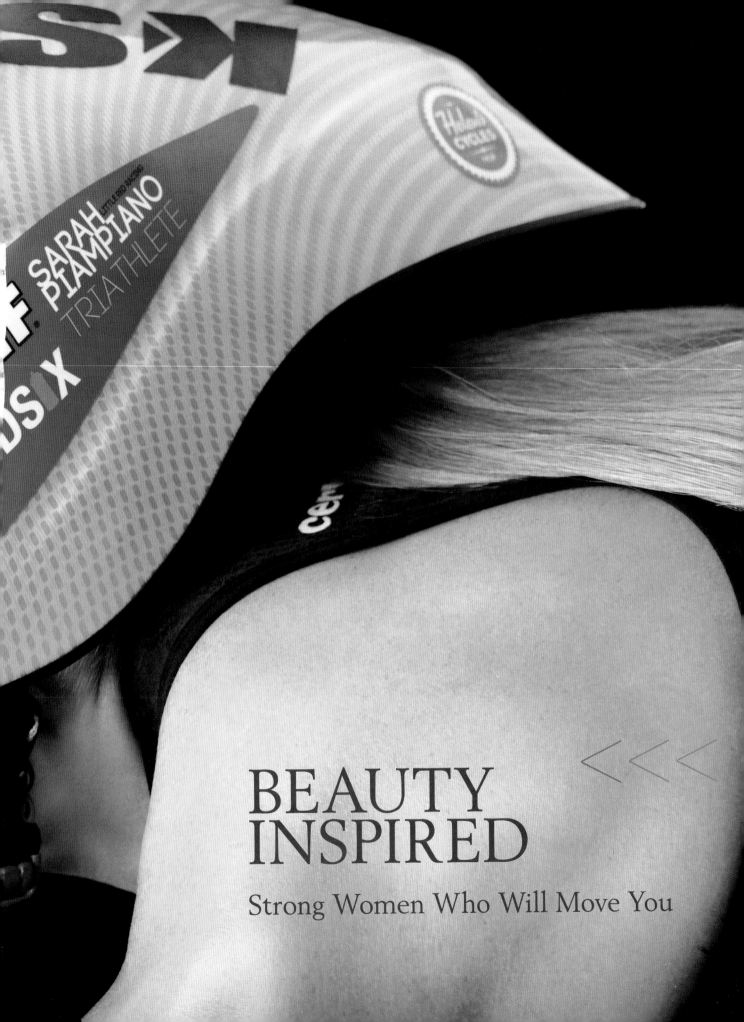

SARAH PIAMPIANO
LITTLE RED MACHINE
TRIATHLETE

BEAUTY INSPIRED

Strong Women Who Will Move You

‹‹‹

Karen Aydelott

NAME: Karen Aydelott

AGE: A proud (but difficult to believe—when did I become this old?) 67 with the wrinkles, lines, and scars to prove it!

OCCUPATION: Volunteer/amateur triathlete

DESCRIBE YOURSELF: A wife, a mother, a grandmother, a graduate of Wellesley College with a BA in art history. I am a retired YMCA executive who ran Y's in Minneapolis, Pasadena, and San Luis Obispo, and am now an inveterate community volunteer for health, youth development, food policy, and strategic planning. And never a beauty queen! I am also an Ironman triathlete—a successful one for many years—which came as a surprise. I just loved the challenge and the sense of accomplishment racing provided. That has just increased now that I race as a below-the-knee amputee. I have amazing role models among the many challenged athletes who have overcome so much more than I have.

WHAT INSPIRES YOU? Opportunities to make a positive difference and to do and be the best that I can.

WHAT BRINGS YOU JOY? Family, friends, and the beauty of the world around me; the sense of accomplishment of a "job" well done.

I FEEL MY BEST WHEN: Everything feels right; also when I am cycling, running, or swimming . . .

MY BEAUTY ICON: Audrey Hepburn, for her classic style, grace, and beauty; for her belief that beauty comes from within; and for all her wonderful philanthropic work.

I CAN'T LIVE WITHOUT: Sunblock and a touch of eyeliner—oh, and my beautiful carbon fiber leg!

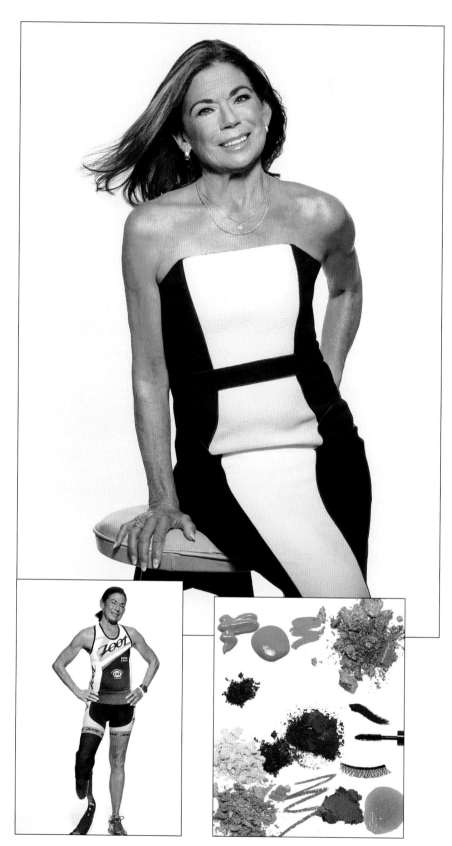

Prep skin by washing face with a gentle cleanser. Massage hydrating lotion into the skin. Repeat one or two times until skin feels plump. Apply eye cream, lip treatment, serum, moisturizer, and sunscreen.

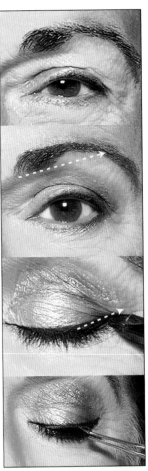

SKIN

1. Apply a medium-beige sheer fluid foundation all over the face and neck.
2. Contour using a tan sheer foundation to the outside edges of the face, the temples, the cheeks, and sides of the nose; and under the jawline, neck, and chest.
3. Apply ocher concealer under eyes, and on bridge of the nose and chin.
4. Set foundation using a translucent loose powder.
5. Apply bronzer along the cheekbones and temples as well as along the hairline.
6. Apply a warm pink blush at the apples of the cheeks.

EYES

1. Apply a shimmering opal base eye shadow to the base of the lids and along the bottom lash lines and inner corners to widen and open up eyes.
2. Apply dark-ash-brown contour eye shadow to the outside corners of the eyes, angling up to lift eyes and apply above the crease.
3. Apply a second layer of contour eye shadow along the outside corners of the lower lash lines to widen eyes.
4. Apply black cream eyeliner along the top of the lash lines. Start thin and thicken the line while extending up at a 45-degree angle at the outside corners of the eyes.

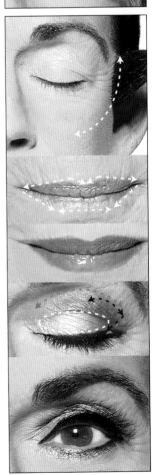

LASHES

1. Curl eyelashes at the base, middle, and tips.
2. Apply two coats of black mascara to the top and bottom lashes.
3. Apply full-strip soft-volume false lashes to lift eyes up.

BROWS

1. Apply medium-ash-brown brow powder along the tops of brows and lightly fill in the sparse areas. Apply a dark brown brow powder to the tails and fill in a thin line from beginning of brow to arch.

LIPS

1. Apply warm brown lip liner slightly outside the natural lip line.
2. Apply warm rose cream lipstick to the entire mouth, covering the lip liner.
3. Apply sheer peach lip gloss to the center of the mouth.

Alexandra Paul

NAME: Alexandra Paul

AGE: 50

OCCUPATION: Environmentalist/Actor

DESCRIBE YOURSELF: Twin, vegan, in love with Ian, athlete, environmentalist, actress, chatterer, nonfiction reader, crossworder, Hallie's mom.

I AM INSPIRED BY: People with passion and purpose.

I AM HAPPIEST WHEN: Walking outside, swimming in warm clear ocean water, being with Ian, snuggling with our kitty, laughing with my mom, or talking with my twin.

I FEEL MY BEST WHEN: I am eating well, working out a lot, busy with work, and going to bed every night with my husband.

MY BEAUTY ICON: Jane Fonda

I CAN'T LIVE WITHOUT: Beauty-wise: brown or gray pencil. Heart-wise: Ian and my sister. Everything-else-wise: being active.

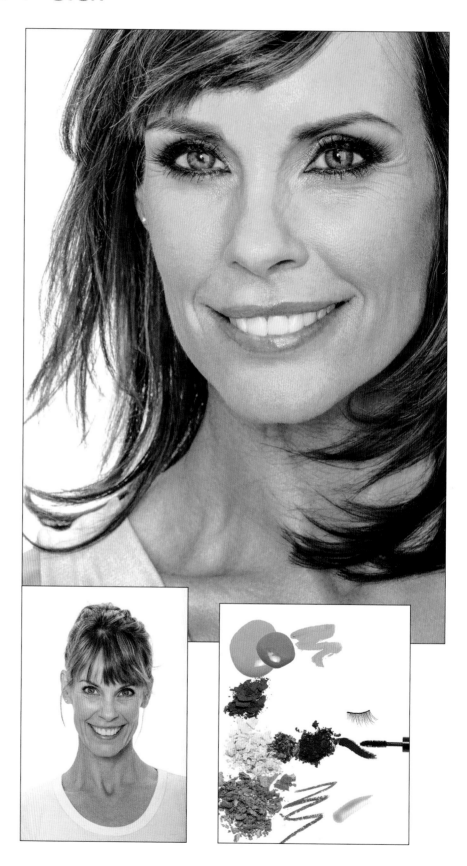

SKIN

1. Apply a thin layer of beige fluid foundation all over the face and neck.
2. Contour using tan fluid foundation to the outside edges of the face, the temples, the cheeks, sides of the nose, and under the jawline.
3. Apply a light application of pink blush at the apples of the cheeks.

EYES

1. Apply shimmering opal eye shadow to the base of the lids, inner corners, and along the bottom lash lines.
2. Apply bronze eye shadow to the outside corners of the eyes and into the creases.
3. Apply dark brown eye shadow to the outside corners of the eyes.
4. Apply black cream eyeliner along the top lash lines and at a 45-degree angle at the outside corners of the eyes and along the lower lash lines.
5. Apply waterproof eyeliner in the waterline.

LASHES

1. Curl eyelashes at the base, middle, and tips.
2. Apply two coats of volumizing black mascara to the top and bottom lashes.
3. Apply short half black false eyelashes to the outside corners of the eyes.

BROWS

1. Apply light-ash-brown eyebrow powder along the tops of brows and lightly fill in the sparse areas. Extend the tails of the brows.

LIPS

1. Apply dark-nude lip liner slightly above the natural lip line.
2. Apply sheer pink lip gloss to the entire mouth.

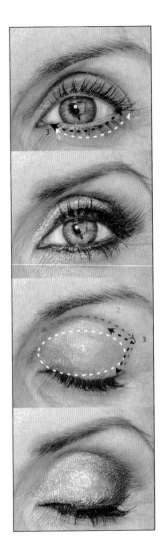

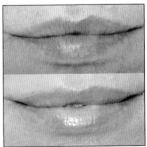

Sarah Piampiano

NAME: Sarah Piampiano

AGE: 33

OCCUPATION: professional triathlete

DESCRIBE YOURSELF: I'm an ex–investment banker and two-pack-a-day cigarette smoker turned professional triathlete; I'm a sister to two brothers; an aunt to four nieces; a wine, ice cream, and cheeseburger lover; I am an aspiring surfer; and an ex–ski racer. I love adventure and the outdoors—hiking, camping, skiing, swimming, boating, sky diving, water skiing; I love to travel; I'm a dog lover, but cat hater; my biggest fear is letting people down.

I AM INSPIRED BY: People who live their life to the fullest; who are independent and strong yet place a high value on relationships; who can be vulnerable with confidence; who aren't afraid to fail; who are modest; people who love life and all of the challenges and adventures it brings and seem to navigate it all with ease, grace and kindness; people who have turned negative events or situations in their lives into positives; dreamers.

I AM HAPPIEST WHEN: Running down a country road on a clear, crisp, fall day; riding my bike along the ocean; being with the people I love most in life; the sense of accomplishment that comes with Ironman racing; waking up every morning next to the love of my life; my nieces; road trips with great music; Sweet Rose ice cream; dreaming big; being a hopeless romantic; being at our family cabin in Maine.

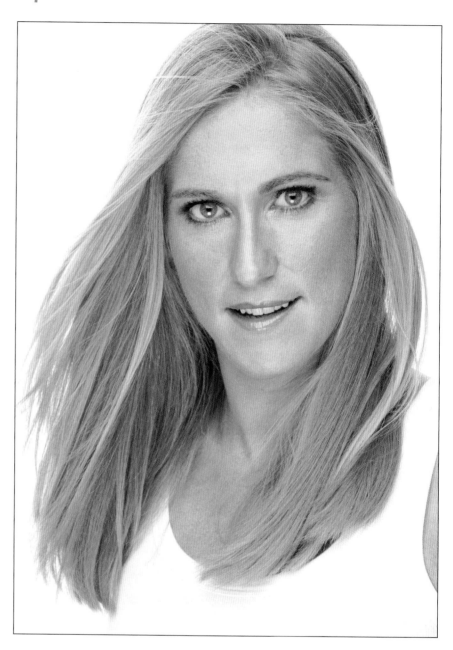

I FEEL MY BEST WHEN: I'm healthy, fit, in a place that I love and with people I love more.

MY BEAUTY ICON: Gwyneth Paltrow. She has an amazing way of putting together looks that are sophisticated and timeless, but edgy and modern. I admire her style and look, and her personality, which is confident and self-assured.

I CAN'T LIVE WITHOUT: Music; my water bottle; my running shoes; a good pair of sunglasses; my gold necklace with a "cherished love" charm.

Look 1

SKIN

1. Apply a natural beige cream foundation all over the face and neck.
2. Contour using a tan stick cream foundation to the outside edges of the face, the temples, the cheeks, sides of the nose and under the jawline.
3. Apply beige concealer under the eyes.
4. Set foundation using translucent loose powder.
5. Apply golden-brown bronzer along the cheekbones and temples.
6. Apply soft pink blush at the apples of the cheeks.

EYES

1. Apply taupe shimmering highlighter base to the base of the lids and along the bottom lash lines and inner corners.
2. Apply warm brown shimmering contour eye shadow to the outside corners of the eyes, slightly above the crease and along outside bottom lash lines.
3. Apply black cream eyeliner along the top three-quarters of the lash line and at a 45-degree angle at the outside corners of the eyes.

LASHES

1. Curl eyelashes at the base, middle, and tips.
2. Apply two coats of black mascara to the top and bottom lashes.
3. Apply individual short black eyelashes to the outside corners of the eyes.

BROWS

1. Apply taupe-brown brow powder along the tops of brows and lightly fill in the sparse areas.
2. Apply heavier application to the tails of the brows.

LIPS

1. Apply natural lip liner slightly above the natural lip line.
2. Apply pinky-beige sheer lip gloss to the center of the mouth.

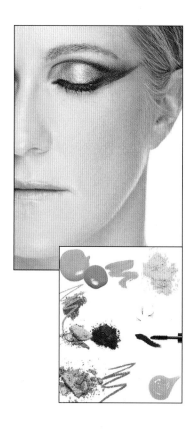

Look 2

SKIN

1. Apply a natural beige cream foundation all over the face and neck.
2. Contour using a tan stick cream foundation to the outside edges of the face, the temples, the cheeks, sides of the nose, and under the jawline.
3. Apply beige concealer under the eyes.
4. Set foundation using translucent loose powder.
5. Apply golden-brown bronzer along the cheekbones and temples.
6. Apply soft pink blush at the apples of the cheeks.

EYES

1. Apply shimmering silver eye shadow to the base of the lids and into the inner corners of the eyes.
2. Extend the silver into the temples and outer corners of the eyes.
3. Apply black eye shadow in a fish shape by extending the outer corners of the eyes. Apply into the creases and bring down to the inner corner of the eyes slightly above the crease and along outside bottom lash lines.
4. Apply black cream eyeliner along the lash lines and at a 45-degree angle at the outside corners of the eyes.
5. Apply bright pink eye shadow under the extended liner and onto the cheekbone.

LASHES

1. Curl eyelashes at the base, middle, and tips.
2. Apply two coats of black mascara to the top and bottom lashes.
3. Apply individual short black eyelashes to the outside corners of the eyes.

BROWS

1. Apply taupe-brown brow powder along the tops of brows and lightly fill in the sparse areas.
2. Apply heavier application to the tails of the brows.

LIPS

1. Apply natural lip liner slightly above the natural lip line.
2. Apply pinky-beige sheer lip gloss to the center of the mouth.

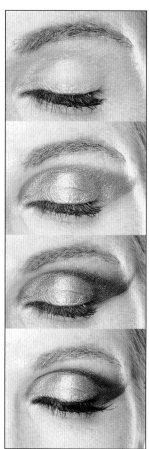

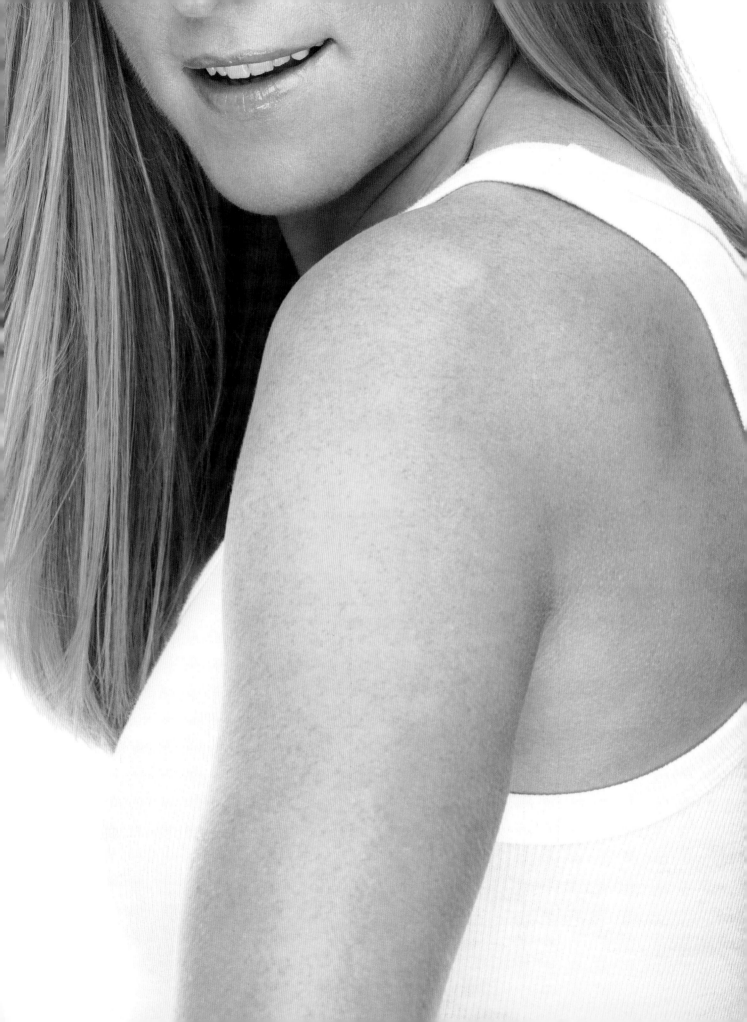

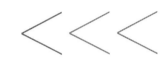

BODY REWIND

Getting Active

think one of the best things I did as I got older was get active. I had been a couch potato and never ran even a mile. I was too busy and too tired and had a million other excuses. Once you decide that you want to take better care of yourself, you can turn the clock back on your body, but most important, you will feel better about yourself. You don't have to do a marathon or triathlon. Everyday choices—such as eating lean protein, working out with heavier weights, or taking walks to keep your body moving—will help slow down the aging process. Our bodies are amazing: The more you move them, the more they can do. Keep your body active so you can continue to be strong and healthy into the late stages of your life.

What do you need to run?
A body, and a desire to do so.

—David Levine

As I got closer to forty, I started to reassess my life. I had already accomplished a lot of what I'd wanted to achieve in my career. I had two kids and a long, happy marriage, but for some reason I still wasn't content. I racked my brain to figure it out. I had what most people thought was everything, but what I realized was that there was too much output and nothing coming in. I did what most women do: take care of everyone and everything else and put myself last. I hadn't taken a vacation for twenty years, not even a honeymoon. I had taken only three weeks off after having each child and still worked from home. What I ended up with was pure exhaustion.

The one good thing about coming close to a breakdown was that I was finally ready to take care of me. There was no guilt involved (okay, maybe some) and I made a list of what I wanted. At the top of that list was that I didn't want to be tired anymore. I had let my physical and mental health go. I was overweight, and diets only last so long. In fact, when I dieted it only made things worse because yet again I had to give something up; besides, I needed food to keep myself going since I worked constantly. So I tried something new. I stopped thinking about what I weighed and focused on my mental health and building my body's endurance. The reality was I still had a lot on my plate and none of it was going away—nor did I want it to. I had worked my whole life to have such a full plate and was blessed to have it. I once read "Don't pray for an easier life. Pray for strength to be able to endure the one you have and more."

So I started to run. I chose running because a friend told me it creates clarity in thinking and that's what I needed. This was not an easy decision; I was a high school track dropout. This time around, I started on the treadmill, a minute at a time, really slowly. My focus was only to run longer than the week before, and sure enough, my food intake changed. I noticed how the good food affected my endurance in a positive way, and that I felt sluggish and my performance suffered when I ate poorly.

My husband had bad knees but wanted to work out with me. He couldn't run in the beginning and asked me instead to bike with him. I had never biked before, either; I was terrified of it but wanted to support his exercise efforts. So I pulled out the only bike I had, which was the one my son had when he was seven, to see if I could do it. I endured a bad five miles but felt exhilarated. I had worked so much, my whole life, I had forgotten what it was like to play. When I shared the story of my newfound youth with a friend she said, "Why don't you do a triathlon? I'm training for one now." The idea of a triathlon piqued my curiosity, but I wasn't a strong swimmer. I had dropped out of the swim team, too, when I was six (in case you couldn't tell by now, I wasn't much of an athlete).

I did some research and began to train for my first triathlon. What I did not know was that the race would change my life. Something happened to me in this process—which took about ten months from running my first full mile to finishing my first sprint triathlon, to six months later completing my first marathon. It wasn't my day-to-day life that was different, it was my perception of life. I felt strong. My mental health was improving along with my physical health. Now, I'm not saying everyone should get up and go do a triathlon, but what I am saying is that you should move, for your mental and physical health. Do something that makes you feel strong and you enjoy. Our lives are filled with enough work. Find something that makes you feel like you're playing. Join a club or a team. Change your focus to happiness and health.

YOUR FIRST 5K

David A. Levine is the coauthor of the *Complete Idiot's Guide to Marathon Training* and a certified coach, level 2, with USA Track & Field, and a certified coach, level 1, with USA Triathlon, as well as a coach for USA Marathon Training and the L.A. Running Club.

How should you begin running if you've never run before?

For any distance, start with low intensity. Yes, it can reduce the risk of injury, but the real reason is that there are certain internal functions that make you more efficient and that you receive only at low levels of intensity. Specifically, you develop capillary veins and arteries, the smallest veins and arteries going in and out of the muscle. This is critical, as you can get more oxygen and nutrients into the muscle faster and waste product out faster. You also gain more and expanded mitochondria. Mitochondria reside in every cell of your body and generate fuel for the muscles. So essentially, the more you have the more fuel you can generate. There are also myriad other internal functions that you also gain from exercise at any level, but start at a low intensity.

Notice I don't mention the words *fast* or *slow*. These are all relative to uphill climbs, heat, wind, and fatigue. All those things will raise your heart rate and increase your intensity levels.

What if I don't feel like I have the energy to walk. How can I run?

You should not feel as if you have to run. Just get out there and walk. After a time, with consistent training, and more volume, you can do a short run with intervals of walking. With more volume you may eventually be able to run without walking. But again, all exercise should start at low intensity. If running is too high an intensity level to sustain or raises your heart rate too much, then walking is the better choice. Besides, you utilize more fat at low levels of intensity.

Can anyone run?

Yes, anyone can run. But there are conditions where if you run, you may be injured. If you have weak or tight muscles, are very overweight, or suffer from a chronic health condition, you would stand a higher risk of injury.

How much should you train before signing up for your 5K?

It really depends on the individual and what you want to accomplish. If you simply want to finish a 5K, a worthy and often difficult thing to do, you need at least three to four weeks of consistent, low-intensity work. I recommend at least three days a week of training per week.

Is it better to start on the treadmill, track, or street?

If it is dark or you live in a bad neighborhood, start on a treadmill, if you have one available. A track can allow you points of reference. In other words, if you are just beginning a running regimen, you could run the straightaways at low intensity and then walk the curves. I if you don't have a track, or treadmill, however, the street works great. A treadmill works slightly different muscles than running outside does. Rarely have I heard of a 5K on a track, so you will be a touch faster on your 5K by running on land rather than a treadmill. On the other hand, professional athletes do train on treadmills in the winter, so they do work well.

What do you need to run?

A body, and a desire to do so. Beyond that, it's beneficial if you're flexible, and have some strength in the upper-body, core, and leg muscles. You'll also need proper shoes purchased from a specialty running store, and not just the cool-looking shoes from a sports store. Running clothes are also a plus. Cotton weighs you down with sweat. Running naked can be fun, but it's a bit drafty. Instead, opt for running clothes with moisture-wicking fabric.

How much should you increase your running week by week?

No more than about 10 to 15 percent. And never add intensity (higher heart rate work), without first dropping volume.

Is running for everyone, at any age?

Anyone can build up to it. But not everyone is ready to go out and start running. Walking is for most people. Age is not the issue here. There was a man who finished a marathon last year and was one hundred years old. I knew a ninety-three-year-old who finished the LA Marathon. Running can be for anyone, however, if you properly prepare yourself for it first. Depending on the individual, this generally takes some stretching and strength training first. And in most adult cases, runners need to learn better form and how to run. Many runners I have worked with on form find they can enjoy running way more once they have learned how to do it properly.

Have fun out there! That's the key!

YOGA

Mandy Ingber is a celebrity fitness expert and *New York Times* bestselling author of *Yogalosophy: 28 Days to the Ultimate Mind-Body Makeover.* Her eighteen years of experience have attracted clients such as Jennifer Aniston, Kate Beckinsale, Brooke Shields, and Helen Hunt.

What is yoga?

Traditionally yoga is the set of disciplines and philosophy that originated in the East to aid practitioners in finding peace. The word *yoga* means "to unite" or "union" and has come to be a form of physical, breathing, and meditation practices that allow the alignment of the heart, mind, body, and spirit. In my opinion, the daily, consistent practice of yoga brings self-acceptance and boosts self-esteem. There is an increased level of self-love and self-care that builds confidence. To me, this is the biggest beauty bonus. When you see a woman who is comfortable in her own skin, balanced and serene (in that she knows she can face difficulty with equanimity), that is beauty. That is one of the main yoga takeaways.

How is yoga helpful in keeping the body young?

The benefits of yoga range from calming the nervous system to controlling weight, improving digestion (which is a key to good health) and circulation, and blood-flow reversal through inversions. The body remains supple and flexible. Being less reactive and less stressed is probably the greatest bonus and benefit to the body and to youth.

How should a beginner start practicing yoga?

A beginner can go to any beginner yoga class. It is usually best to have some personal attention, and get familiar with the poses. Tell the instructor you are new. Start in the back of the room so that you may follow along. There are all different styles of yoga. Iyengar is a great style that focuses on alignment and form. If you want a more stretchy type of yoga, try Yin or Restorative. Yoga has become so mainstream that there is something for everyone. If you like hip-hop music, they have it; surf yoga, yep . . . the list goes on, so try at least six different styles and teachers before deciding if yoga is for you.

What is the best time to practice yoga?

The morning is a wonderful time, as you gather and harness all of the early-morning energy, plus you get to check it off of your to-do list. But whatever time you are able to find is good. I honestly find that people in general are looking for the right and wrong, but you must explore and find what works best for your body, energy level, and schedule.

How often should you be practicing yoga?

There are no "shoulds." Yoga can be a daily practice. I always say to do whatever you are able to maintain on a regular basis. If that's three times a week, great. It is better to do twenty minutes of yoga three times a week, than four hours of yoga once every two weeks. Be consistent.

What are a few key yoga poses that are great for strengthening?

Side angle pose
Tree pose
Triangle
Warrior II

What are a few key yoga poses for stretching?

Forward bend (standing or seated)
Pigeon
Plough
Standing splits

Is there anything I should do before starting a yoga regimen?

Cultivate a sense of patience and curiosity. It really isn't about doing the pose correctly. There is a saying: move a muscle, change a thought. Often we overthink things or can be just plain hard on ourselves because we compare ourselves to other people. Just set aside some time and space for your yoga practice. At first you may have to make yourself do it, then you will simply show up. Soon you will look forward to it . . . and then, watch out! You may just change your schedule to work around your practice! Purchase a sticky mat and wear comfy clothes that won't ride over your head when you're upside down during the practice. Make sure your feet are clean, as you will be barefoot. Always do yoga on a relatively empty stomach. Don't expect to know what you are doing right away. You can always check out a yoga website online to get an orientation to the basics and see what the poses look like.

NUTRITION

Growing up being the "chubby sister" forced me to try pretty much every type of restrictive diet. Limiting calories left me tired and I often failed as body cravings beat will and left me feeling defeated and a few pounds heavier than when I started. It took looking at food as energy to give me perspective.

It's important to view food as fuel, period. Like a car, the more activity you do the more fuel you need; and the better the gas, the better the car's performance. Now imagine that fuel actually will help determine how shiny the car looks, whether or not the color will be vibrant, and the life expectancy of the vehicle. Of course, as we've learned, there are never any guarantees; outside factors such as genetics and environment can shorten this life span, but as you would take care of your home, that much more care you should put in for your health. You can always move homes, but you only get one body. The rule of thumb is to consume as many natural foods as you possibly can, but don't starve yourself and don't eat past being full.

SUGAR

I don't think I've ever met anyone who said they hated sugar! Beyond the health issues—diabetes, heart disease, and a slew of other illnesses—processed sugar as well as refined sugar need to be limited as sugar actually prohibits the growth of collagen. This results in older-looking skin.

WATER

It is important to drink plenty of water to remove the toxins in your body and help it to function properly. Water consumption also helps to curb appetite. Drink six to eight 8-ounce glasses per day, more if you're a caffeine drinker as caffeine dehydrates the body and skin.

GOOD FATS

As we age, our skin produces less oil, which can make it appear dull and dry. Good fats help skin cells work at their optimum level. Eating foods high in omegas help to keep skin glowing and keeps hydration at an optimum. Avocados, fish, and nuts are a great source of good fats.

ANTIOXIDANTS

Feed your cells foods rich in antioxidants so your body can fight free radicals and minimize cell damage. Antioxidant-rich foods include berries, apples, beans, and nuts.

LEAN PROTEIN

Protein is in every part of our body, and eating protein-rich foods is essential to help cells repair themselves. Eggs, skinless chicken, and tofu are great sources of protein to keep the body running at optimum levels. Cottage cheese and Greek yogurts also deliver large amounts of protein.

DARK GREEN VEGETABLES

The darker the vegetable, the more minerals and vitamins you are getting. Since dark veggies, such as kale and spinach, are high in fiber, they'll give you energy and keep you feeling full longer.

STRENGTH AND STRETCH

I clearly remember being at the gym and doing my ten-pound bicep curls when a very fit man came up to me and asked if I was using the twenty-five-pound dumbbells that were on the floor next to me. I looked at him, confused. As if I could ever work with such heavy weights! I wondered if he was joking. Recently, I reached for thirty-pound dumbbells and it reminded me of that moment. Again, I'm not saying you should go work with such heavy weights—at least not at the beginning—but it's yet another reminder that your body can really surprise you.

A muscle will only grow if it needs to grow. If you are working with weights similar to the amount you regularly pick up—for example, the same general heft as your groceries, backpack, or purse—your body will not feel the need to adjust. You need to stress your body to cause it to react. Work with lower reps and higher weights to create muscle growth. You can do this using free weights or doing yoga, which forces you to use your own body weight. Building muscle is important to keep your body strong. Muscle also burns more calories than fat, so muscle is essential to keep your metabolism higher. You can weigh the same but your clothes will fit looser. Most important, keeping muscles from atrophying will help your body stay strong and mobile as you age, and can prevent many injuries such as falling and broken bones.

Stretching is key to keeping your body young, limber, and free from injury. Stretch while lying on the ground as oftentimes after a rigorous workout you can get dizzy standing and bending over to stretch. Focus on stretching your back, the backs of your legs, and hips. Make sure to always be gentle to your muscles when stretching and avoid doing anything aggressively. Like running or any other exercise, it's important to increase flexibility slowly. Avoid jerking and overstretching, which can pull muscles and cause injury.

STYLING

Dos and Don'ts to Look Younger

Named one of the most powerful stylists in Hollywood by the *Hollywood Reporter*, Jeanne Yang began her career as managing editor and associate publisher at *Detour* magazine. Jeanne's talent and foresight put then unknowns from Leonardo DiCaprio to Sandra Bullock to Cameron Diaz on covers. Her photo credits include covers and editorials for *GQ*, *InStyle*, *Vanity Fair*, *Rolling Stone*, and *Vogue*.

What are some styling mistakes that make women look much older than they are? Why?

One of the biggest mistakes you can make at any age is trying to be so trend-conscious and not acknowledging what works best on your body. Being a fashion victim is a surefire way of revealing your age, making you look silly. For example, it is always best to try jeans that are the most flattering to your particular body type, even if skinny jeans are what are happening right now.

When do you know it's time to throw things out?

When the fabric is pilled and faded or falling apart, there is not much you can do to rescue a piece. Try to invest in better-quality pieces and look for clothing made from natural fibers and smaller stitches. These are telltale signs that something will last longer.

What are the best pieces to invest in?

Stylish women invest in better quality and buy less. Resist the temptation to buy lots of cheap clothing. It is better to get a few great pieces at resale shops or at outlets and at sales.

What jewelry makes bold statements that work? Is less more?

Wearing less but wearing precious or semiprecious stones and gold or silver is a smarter investment. These pieces will maintain their value and can always be melted down and made into new pieces.

What are key pieces that every woman should own to update their wardrobe? Why?

A great black dress, amazing suede pumps, a well-tailored white shirt, and a pair of flattering jeans. Avoid the baggy, ripped-up pair, and pick up a dark rinse jean you can wear to almost any event. And invest in a great trench or longer coat. It is the first thing people see when they meet you.

What is the proper footwear for aging feet?

Insoles solve so many issues. First make sure you have well-fitting shoes. Then buy some insoles with an arch or some cushion. The comfort factor will make most any shoe wearable.

What pieces elongate and slim the body?

Monochromatic head-to-toe or looks with contrasting sides in black can cut a nice, slim silhouette. Typically, a higher-waisted pair of pants or dress can create a longer leg.

What's the proper skirt length?

Hold up the skirt and slowly raise it up your leg. You will be able to see where to hem the length of any skirt or dress to ensure it is the most flattering bottom for your body type.

What pieces should you invest in and what pieces can you get away with spending less on?

Coats, sweaters, and shirts are more important as people will notice these more than pants, and poor quality is hard to hide in a cheaply made coat or sweater. Pants can be skimped on a little bit as they will get more wear.

100 QUICK TIPS

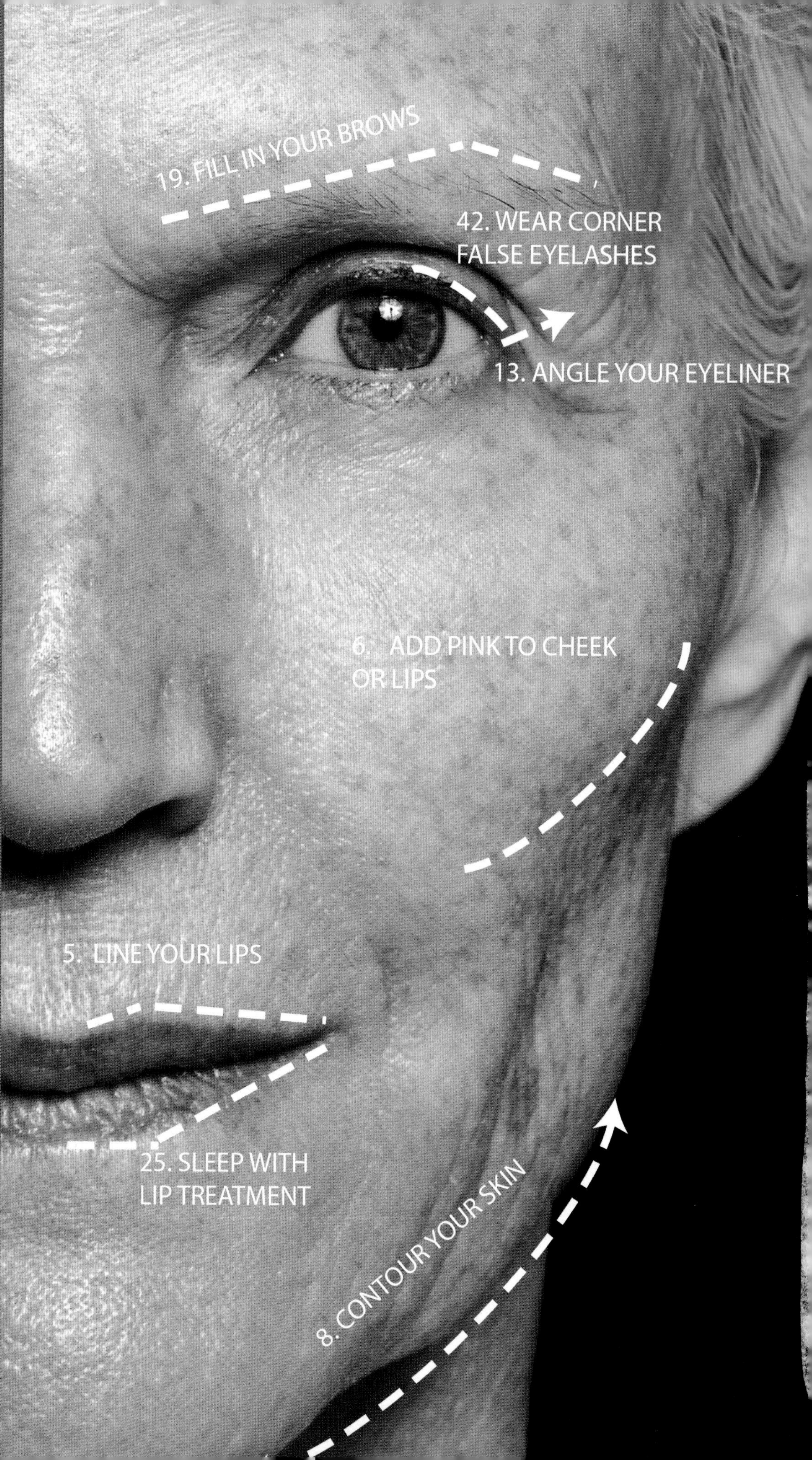

19. FILL IN YOUR BROWS

42. WEAR CORNER
FALSE EYELASHES

13. ANGLE YOUR EYELINER

6. ADD PINK TO CHEEK
OR LIPS

5. LINE YOUR LIPS

25. SLEEP WITH
LIP TREATMENT

8. CONTOUR YOUR SKIN

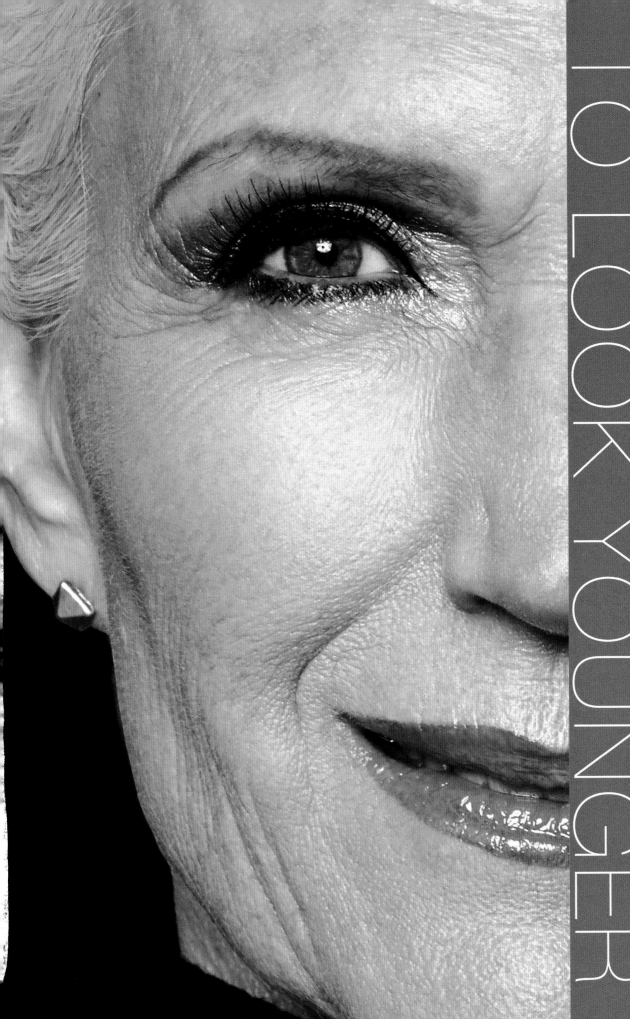

TO LOOK YOUNGER

1. Brighten your hair color

2. Whiten your teeth

3. Soften your haircut

4. Incorporate a face serum into your skin-care routine

5. Line your lips

6. Add pink to your cheeks or lips

7. Change your perfume

8. Contour your skin

9. Use body makeup

10. Curl your lashes

11. Minimize bottom eyeliner

12. Brighten your eye shadow

13. Angle your eyeliner

14. Wear contour eye shadow

15. Wear black mascara

16. Wear shape wear

17. Shorten your nails

18. Wear modern nail colors

19. Fill in your brows

20. Darken your foundation

21. Exfoliate your skin

22. Wear eye cream morning and night

23. Wear eye-treatment pads twice a week

24. Soften your blush

25. Sleep with lip treatment

26. Use retinol-based night cream

27. Use sunscreen SPF 30+

28. Start your eyebrows with a lighter color and darken tails

29. Toss out dated panty hose

30. Use waterproof liners and mascaras

31. Use less powder

32. Prime eyelids with foundation

33. Avoid tight or baggy clothing

34. Invest in shoes

35. Invest in handbags

36. Soften your brow bone

37. Wear lip gloss

38. Wear sunglasses

39. Use hand cream

40. Add dimension to your hair with highlights or lowlights

41. Use makeup on your chest

42. Wear corner false eyelashes

43. Wear cream blush

44. Use face highlighter

45. Use beige liner inside your waterline

46. Add shimmer

47. Smile

48. Control the shine

49. Switch up your skin care

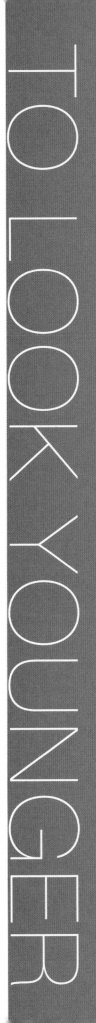

TO LOOK YOUNGER

50. Break a sweat

51. Use a treatment mask twice a week

52. Do a cleanse

53. Limit white sugar

54. Cover up hyperpigmentation

55. Practice pressure-point massage

56. Remove excess facial hair

57. Reshape your brows

58. Massage your face

59. Steam your face

60. Use bronzer

61. Use makeup brushes

62. Meditate or pray

63. Apply concealer after foundation

64. Exfoliate daily

65. Wear colors in the same family

66. Waterproof your eye makeup

67. Add vitamin C

68. Moisturize daily

69. Get seven to nine hours' sleep every night

70. Take essential vitamins daily

71. Use satin or silk pillowcases

72. Take care of your scalp

73. Start the day by doing something nice for yourself

74. Keep skin-care products by your bed

75. Bathe in essential oils

76. Switch to tea

77. Minimize caffeine

78. Drink more water

79. Apply thicker liner on the top lash line as opposed to the bottom lash line

80. Update your bras

81. Don't rub your eyes

82. Use eye makeup remover

83. Don't touch your face

84. Change your hair part

85. Breathe deeply, counting to ten

86. Eat good fats such as olive oil and avocado

87. Take vitamin D

88. Update your eyeglass frames

89. Conceal dark circles

90. Fill in your pores using primer or foundation

91. Pluck, don't wax, your brows

92. Add shimmer to your eye shadows

93. Sleep on your back

94. Eat good carbs such as yams

95. Work out with weights

96. Brighten your wardrobe

97. Practice good posture

98. Do short-burst exercises

99. Eat more lean protein

100. Change your shampoo

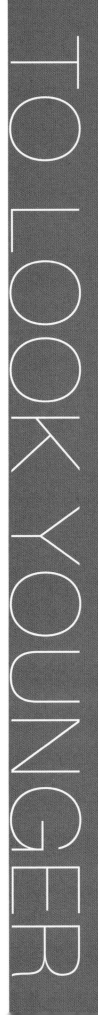

TO LOOK YOUNGER

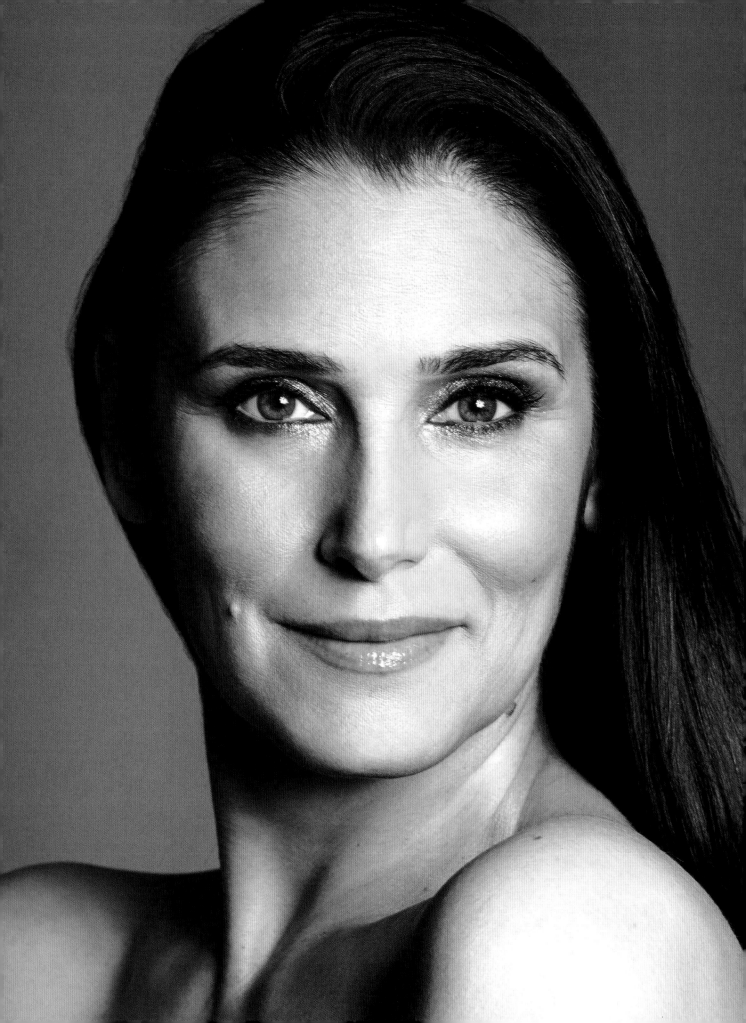

RESOURCES

Go to beautyrewind.com for updates on resource guide

FOLLOW TAYLOR:

 TWITTER: ©taylorbabaian

 FACEBOOK: taylor babaian

PRODUCTS

COSMETICS, SKIN CARE, AND TOOLS

Anastasia (Anastasia.net) cosmetics for eyes and brows

Aquaphor Healing Ointment (aquaphorhealing.com) skin care, moisturizers

Armani Beauty (giorgioarmanibeauty-usa.com) cosmetics

Avon (avon.com) cosmetics, skin care

Bare Escentuals (Bareescentuals.com) mineral makeup

Benefit (Benefitcosmetics.com) brow bars and cosmetics

blinc (blincinc.com) cosmetics for eyes

Bobbi Brown Cosmetics (bobbibrowncosmetics.com) cosmetics

By Terry (byterry.com) cosmetics

Chanel (chanel.com) cosmetics, skin care

Clarisonic (clarisonic.com) exfoliating brushes

Clé de Peau Beauté (cledepeau-beaute.com/en; facebook.com/
 cledepeaubeauteus) luxury skin care, foundations, cosmetics

Clinique (Clinique.com) cosmetics, skin care

Colorescience (colorescience.com) mineral makeup

Crest (3dwhite.com) tooth whitening strips

Dermablend (dermablend.com) face, leg, and body cover

Dermalogica (dermalogica.com) skin care (offers free Face Mapping* skin
 analysis and guests can obtain free samples of products)

Dr. Jessica Wu (drjessicawu.com)

Eau Thermale Avene (aveneusa.com) sensitive skin care, thermal spring water

Ecotools (ecotools.com) brushes, puffs

Elizabeth Arden (Elizabetharden.com) skin care, cosmetics, bodycare

Essie (essie.com) nail color

Estée Lauder (esteelauder.com) cosmetics, skin care

Eucerin (eucerinus.com) sensitive skin care products

Heir Atelier (heiratelier.com) skin prep

Hourglass Makeup (hourglasscosmetics.com) cosmetics and brushes

Kevyn Aucoin (kevynaucoin.com) cosmetics and brushes

Krē•at Beauty (kreatbeauty.com) prestige false eyelashes and tools

L'Oreal Paris (lorealparisusa.com) cosmetics, hair and skin care

Lancôme (lancome-usa.com) skin care and cosmetics

Laura Mercier (lauramercier.com) cosmetics

LORAC (loraccosmetics.com) cosmetics

MAC Cosmetics (maccosmetics.com) cosmetics

Make Up For Ever (makeupforever.com) brushes, cosmetics

Mary Kay (marykay.com) cosmetics

Maybelline (maybelline.com) cosmetics, mascaras

Merle Norman Cosmetics (merlenorman.com) cosmetics

Murad (murad.com) skin care products

NARS Cosmetics (narscosmetics.com) cosmetics

Neutrogena (neutrogena.com) sunscreens, skin care, cosmetics

Nioxin (nioxin.com) hair-loss treatment

Olay (olay.com) exfoliating brushes, skin care

Red Carpet Kolour (redcarpetkolour.com) body shimmers

Rembrandt (rembrant.com) tooth whiteners

Revlon (revlon.com) cosmetics

Rogaine (rogaine.com) hair-loss treatment

Rubistweezers (rubistweezers.com)

Seche vite (seche.com) long-wear topcoat for nails

Sephora (sephora.com) products, videos

Shiseido (shiseido.com) complimentary facial services available at Shiseido nationwide

Sonia Kashuk (soniakashuk.com) cosmetics, brushes

St tropez (sttropeztan.com) body bronzers, shimmers, conditioners

Stila Cosmetics (stilacosmetics.com) cosmetics

Tom Ford (tomford.com) cosmetics

Toppik (toppik.com) hair building fibers

Troy Surrat (surrattbeauty.com) cosmetics

Tweezerman (tweezerman.com) eyebrow tools

Vanity Mark (vanitymark.com) cosmetics and tools, brow bar, body bronzers

Ziba Beauty (zibabeauty.com) brow bars

DEPARTMENT STORES

FOR MAKEUP SERVICES AND THE LATEST PRODUCTS. CALL AHEAD FOR OFFERS AND APPOINTMENTS.

Barneys New York (barneys.com)

Bergdorf Goodman (bergdorfgoodman.com)

Bloomingdale's (bloomingdales.com)

Dillard's (dillards.com)

Macy's (macys.com)

Neiman Marcus (neimanmarcus.com)

Nordstrom (nordstrom.com)

Saks Fifth Avenue (saksfifthavenue.com)

Space NK (spacenk.com)

DRUGSTORES

Target (target.com)

Walmart (walmart.com)

Duane Reade (duanereade.com)

Walgreens (walgreens.com)

Ulta (ulta.com)

CVS Pharmacy (cvs.com)

MAGAZINES

Allure (allure.com)

Fitness (fitnessmagazine.com)

MORE (moremagazine.com)

New Beauty Magazine (newbeauty.magazines.com)

Prevention magazine (prevention.com)

Redbook (redbook.com)

Women's Health (womenshealthmag.com)

VIDEOS

Beautyrewind.com

Popsugar.com

Totalbeauty.com

PROFESSIONAL SERVICES

American Academy of Dermatology (aad.org)

American Dental Association (ada.org)

American Society of Plastic Surgeons (plasticsurgery.org)

FITNESS

Soulcycle indoor cycling full-body workout (soul-cycle.com; all first-time riders $20)

Yoga

    Mandy Ingber (mandyingber.com for a free audio download)

    YogaWorks (yogaworks.com)

    Active.com (find fitness events nationwide)

    USA Marathon Training (usamarathontraining.com)

    Runningintheusa.com (running clubs)

    Usatriathlon.org

    Ironman.com (information on ironman distance triathlons)

    Fitness.com/find_gym

VEGAN PRODUCTS

Andalou Naturals (andalou.com)

Artiba Cosmetics (artibacosmetics.com)

JĀSÖN (jason-personalcare.com)

ZuZu Luxe (gabrielcosmeticsinc.com)

GET ACTIVE FOR A CAUSE

ACTIVE (active.com)

Alzheimer's Association (alz.org)

American Heart Association (heart.org)

Autism Speaks—Walk for Autism (autismspeaks.org)

Avon Walk for Breast Cancer (avonwalk.org)

Challenged Athletes Foundation (challengedatletes.org)

EIF Revlon Run/Walk for Women (revlonrunwalk.org)

Pancreatic Cancer Action Network (purplestride.org)

Parkinson's Foundation (pdf.org)

Team in Training (teamintraining.org)

ACKNOWLEDGMENTS

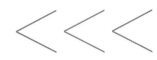

Books are never a one-person job. It literally takes a village to complete one, especially a book of this magnitude. One of the greatest rewards of writing a book is here where I get the opportunity to thank the people who made it possible. It's my Oscar speech and my chance to say a few words of heartfelt gratitude. I never go a day without feeling blessed to have the amazing support around me.

First and foremost, I would like to thank God for all of His blessings. I am grateful for the past, good and bad, which has made me who I am today. This is my third book stating this; the older I get, the more true this has become.

Many thanks also to my family, who brings me sheer joy, laughter, and strength. To my husband, Raffi, my cycling buddy, my marathon partner, and my best friend: Thank you for being a true husband. Your support for every crazy act I think of and your helpfulness during the execution makes everything possible. We have had it hard and grown so much together, and I can't wait to see what lies ahead for us. To my daughter, Adina, I am so proud of the woman you have become. Your passion for your beliefs has been evident even since you were a toddler. Your desire to learn everything from history to baking makes me smile from ear to ear, and your compassion for others gives me the greatest source of pride. Thank you for all your help during the process, assisting from makeup to lighting, graphics, and craft services. I love you more than words. To my son, Christopher: you have grown up to be such a gentleman. You make this mother proud. Thank you for helping me with whatever you could—food delivery, being part of the cleaning crew, or doing heavy lifting—but mostly for the energy and joy you bring with you when you enter a room. Your happiness and positive energy is infectious and will do you well in life. Your acceptance of people for who they are without judgment makes me inspired for the next generation.

To Barbara Sue Smith, a beautiful woman who was mother to all she met, including myself. Thank you for showing me true generosity, for your incredible meals, and, most important, sharing your wise words. Your memory will live in our hearts forever.

To Kobe, my sweet coauthor, you changed my perception of dogs and how a human can love one so much. Thank you for sitting with me year after year, when I had to pull weeks of all-nighters. It was hard to finish this book without you. You will be greatly missed, but always remembered.

To my dear, talented friends Albert Sanchez and Pedro Zalba, I am so grateful to collaborate with you both again on yet another great project. Thank you for bringing your energy, love, and your best. You would think by now I would be used to your genius, but you continue to blow me away time and time again.

To Rob Latour, one of my oldest and dearest friends, thanks for being a part of another book and being so giving of your time, talent, and energy. You have always been there no matter what the request and I will always remember that.

To Manuel Benevides, one of the most talented hairdressers I have ever worked with, thank you for being so generous with your time and for being a dear friend.

To Peter Brown, world traveler and kind soul, I just can't thank you enough for your hard work and dedication to this project. You are a true gentleman and I'm so happy that you are still in my life after all this time.

Ron Eshel: It was a full-circle moment working with you. Thank you for being a part of this project and doing it with such joy.

To my friends and amazing contributors, David Levine, Mandy Ingber, Jeanne Yang, and Dr. Jessica Wu, you are the best of the best and I am beyond honored that you have shared your wealth of knowledge in this very personal project.

My utmost gratitude to all the wonderful women who gave so much of themselves to this book. Your honesty and sharing of your life will inspire others for years to come. Keli Lee, Pam Skaist-Levy, Gela Nash Taylor, Karen Aydelott, Jackie Barton, Lisa Butler, Leza Cruz, Marcela Isaza, Alla Clancy, Sarah Piampiano, Stephanie Liner, Alexandra Paul, Jes Macallan, Maye Musk, Valerie Van Galder, Brighdie Grounds, and Wendy Both, thank you for lending your beautiful selves to this book.

To my lovely editor, Jeanette Shaw: I can't believe this is our third book together. I am so grateful for your support, always lending your talent and your page-by-page guidance. Thank you for helping me to fulfill my dream of teaching all women to create their own beauty. Thank you also to John Duff and everyone at Penguin for yet another incredible opportunity.

To Melissa Flashman, my beautiful literary agent, and everyone at Trident Media Group: Thank you for your invaluable support and for being a part of my story. I feel so blessed to have met you all those years ago.

Thanks to everyone at the Cloutier Remix for your day-to-day work and friendship. Madeline Leonard, you have become such a dear friend to me. Your excitement always gives me renewed strength. To Adrienne Novak, Susanna Burke, Peggi Hager, Ben Ahern, Jeanna Bonello, Gwen Kellet, Libby Anderson, Mardie Glen, Dequita Pettiford and everyone at Cloutier past, present, and future, thanks for your love, friendship, and support.

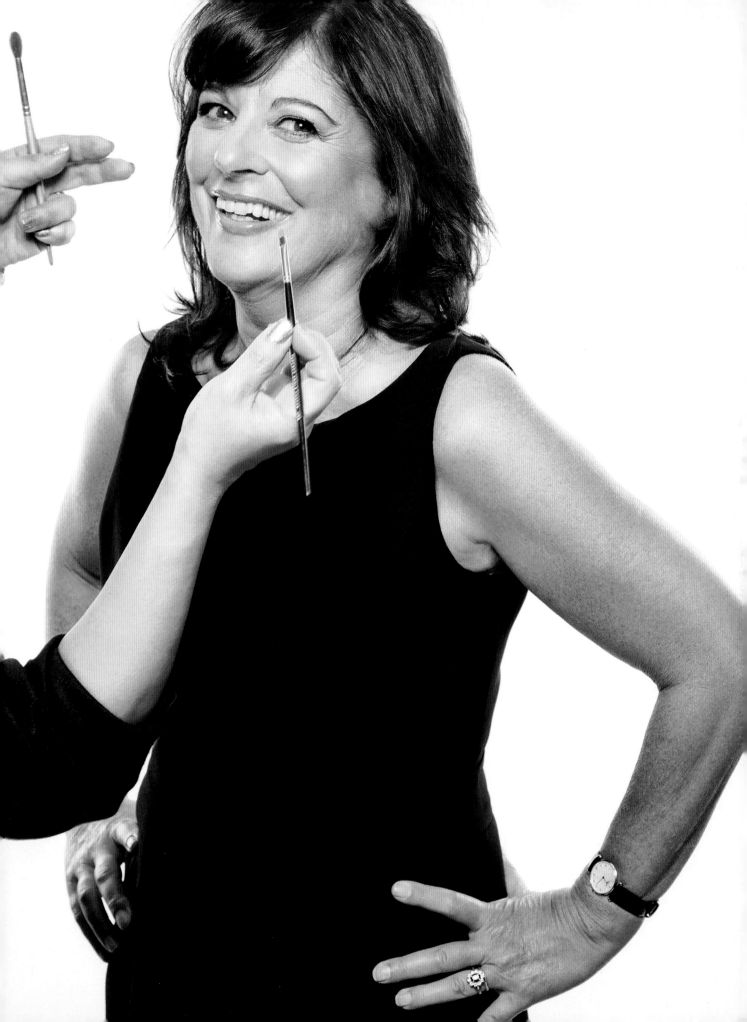

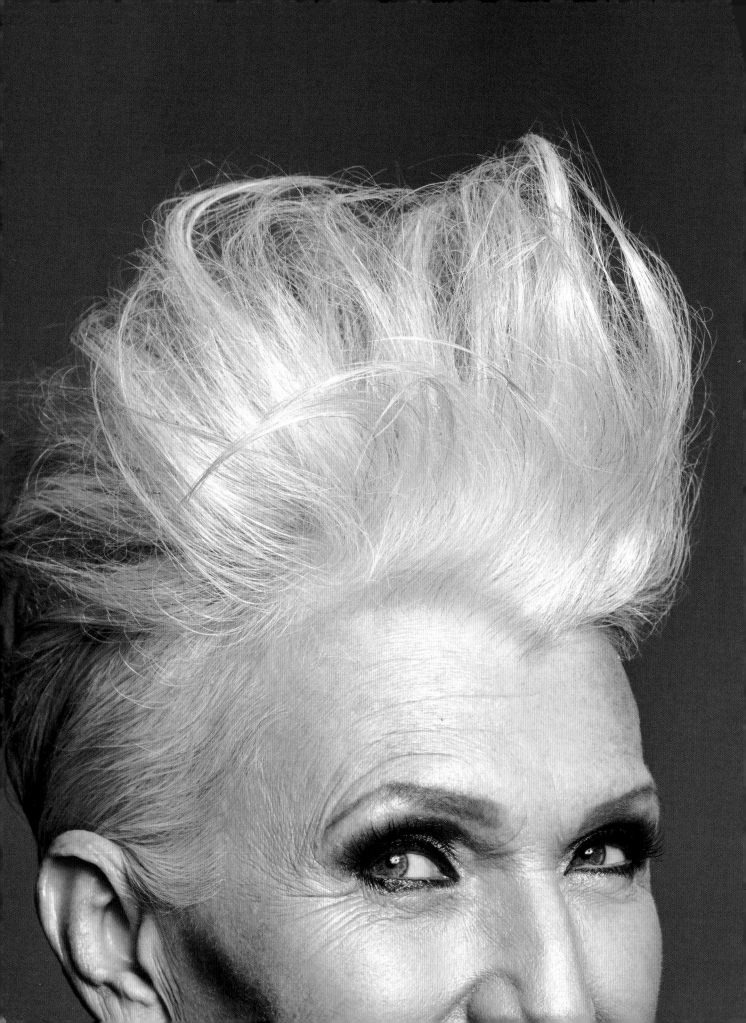

CONTRIBUTORS

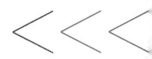

ALBERT SANCHEZ's first foray into image-making was studying photorealist painting in college. He was concurrently experimenting with photography, taking pictures of his glam-rock friends and Barbie Dolls in phantasmagorical scenarios. His career in photography began in earnest in Paris as a portrait photographer and has since expanded into the fields of celebrity portraiture, fashion, and beauty. His notable subjects have included Nicole Kidman, Mick Jagger, and Dita Von Teese, among others. He has shot beauty campaigns for MAC, Revlon, L'Oreal, and Tarina Tarantino Beauty. Drawing on his initial training in airbrushing, Albert enjoys being hands-on in the post production of his photography.

> Pages: iii, v, vi, vii, 8, 14, 30, 39, 46, 49, 51, 52, 55, 62, 65, 74, 102, 120, 121, 122, 128, 130, 160, 161, 166, 174

ROB LATOUR was born and raised in Canada. After a brief stint teaching math, physics, and chemistry the need for a creative balance overpowered logic and he began his professional photography career in Los Angeles, shooting editorial fashion for different magazines ranging from *Teen* magazine to Spanish *Vogue*. He has photographed names such as Jimmy Stewart, Mary Martin, Jack Lemmon, Heidi Klum, Giorgio Armani, George Clooney, Sandra Bullock, and Julie Andrews in his studio and on location. He is currently the West Coast photographer for British *Vogue* online, and has worldwide distribution through Rex Features out of London.

> Pages: xii, 28, 39, 70, 71, 77, 91, 98, 102, 105, 106, 118, 126, 127, 134, 135, 138, 139, 142, 143, 144, 145, 146, 147, 148. All false eyelash photography.

For more than twenty-five years, **PETER BROWN** has remained a standout photographer in fashion, beauty, and the luxury travel circuits. From celebrities and models to entertainment moguls and the lifestyles that follow them, Brown has been there capturing the light every step of the way. He currently resides in Los Angeles, camera in hand. To view more of his work, please visit peterwesleybrown .com.

> Pages: 6, 35, 36, 39, 58, 72, 73, 75, 76, 77, 80, 86, 91, 94, 96, 98, 100, 102, 103, 110, 114, 115, 116, 117, 124, 125, 132, 133, 136, 137, 173

RON ESHEL, a seasoned portrait photographer and director, lives with his wife and twins in Los Angeles. A graduate of London College of Printing, Ron is known for capturing the essence of his subjects using advanced lighting techniques that bring out the elemental beauty of each without pretense or special effects.

Pages: 85, 91, 102, 140, 141. All product photography, excluding eyelashes.

PEDRO ZALBA first began participating on photo shoots as a set designer and prop stylist, working for top photographers such as Herb Ritts and Helmut Newton. For the last decade he has worked exclusively with Albert Sanchez, collaborating on every aspect of image-making from conception through completion.

Pages: iii, v, vi, viii, 8, 14, 30, 39, 46, 49, 51, 52, 55, 62, 65, 74, 102, 120, 121, 122, 128, 130, 160, 161, 166, 174

DAVID A. LEVINE is the coauthor of the *Complete Idiot's Guide to Marathon Training*, part of the international Complete Idiot's series. He has been coaching for ten years, and is currently a certified coach, level 2, with USA Track & Field, and a certified coach, level 1, with USA Triathlon. He coaches USA Marathon Training and the L.A. Running Club.

MANDY INGBER is a celebrity fitness expert and *New York Times* best-selling author of *Yogalosophy: 28 Days to the Ultimate Mind-Body Makeover* (Seal Press), which is available in stores and online at mandyingber.com/yogalosophybook. Her eighteen years of experience have attracted clients such as Jennifer Aniston, Kate Beckinsale, Brooke Shields, and Helen Hunt. She is a keynote speaker, spokesperson, and wellness blogger for People.com and E! Visit Mandy on her website, mandyingber.com, or follow her on Twitter: @msmandyingber, or on Facebook: Mandy Ingber's Yogalosophy.

DR. JESSICA WU is a cosmetic dermatologist practicing in Los Angeles. A graduate of Harvard Medical School, she is assistant clinical professor of dermatology at USC Medical School, and is involved in clinical research trials on injectable and topical antiaging treatments. Dr. Wu recently launched her second skin-care line: Dr. Jessica Wu Skincare, available at Costco stores nationwide. Dr. Wu is a member of the Medical Nutrition Council of the American Society for Nutrition, and is author of *Feed Your Face: Younger, Smoother Skin and a Beautiful Body in 28 Delicious Days*. Dr. Wu shares her passion for helping women live a healthier, beautiful life in her daily e-newsletter, which has more than 150,000 subscribers, and is frequently interviewed on local and national TV shows. Dr. Wu is co-founder of a nonprofit organization, BeautyShares Inc., dedicated to building confidence and self-esteem in disadvantaged teens through workshops that teach grooming and healthy lifestyle choices.

Named one of the most powerful stylists in Hollywood by the *Hollywood Reporter*, **JEANNE YANG** began her career as managing editor and associate publisher at *Detour* magazine. Jeanne's talent and foresight put then unknowns from Leonardo DiCaprio to Sandra Bullock to Cameron Diaz on covers. Jeanne's photo credits include covers and editorials for *GQ*, *InStyle*, *Vanity Fair*, *Rolling Stone*, and *Vogue*. A graduate of Scripps College, she has worked with Hollywood's top A-list actors and continues to consult for major fashion and cosmetic companies on their national advertising campaigns.